Contents

Principles of
SURGERY

*Everything you need to know
but were frightened to ask!*

Sam Andrews
Luke Cascarini

tfm Publishing Limited, Castle Hill Barns, Harley, Nr Shrewsbury, SY5 6LX, UK. Tel: +44 (0)1952 510061; Fax: +44 (0)1952 510192 E-mail: nikki@tfmpublishing.com; Web site: www.tfmpublishing.com

Design & Typesetting: Nikki Bramhill, tfm publishing Ltd.
First Edition: © 2008
Front cover images: © 1999 Image 100 Ltd.
                          © Comstock Inc., www.comstock.com

ISBN: 978 1 903378 57 1

Printed by Gutenberg Press Ltd., Gudja Road, Tarxien, PLA 19, Malta. Tel: +356 21897037; Fax: +356 21800069.

Section 2 The operating theatre environment 71

Foreword

This little book aims to answer the questions that other surgical texts fail to address. Originally designed for junior surgeons with the College of Surgeons' examinations in mind, it is, in fact, essential knowledge on the principles of surgery and operating theatre practice for all healthcare professionals with an interest in surgery.

Surgery is a vast subject with specialists in every area from the podiatrist to the neurosurgeon. What is more, in each operating room there might be many grades and types of health professional: medical or dental student, scrub nurse, junior doctor, operating department assistant and consultant. Each and every one of these groups has their own textbooks. However, there are fundamental facts about surgery which are as relevant to the dental nurse as they are to the professor. This book has been specially compiled to address all these fundamental, pertinent points which everyone who has anything at all to do with surgery should know, but so often actually does not. This book should be read by absolutely anyone who has ever set foot in an operating room or dental surgery; if you don't know what's in this book you probably have no business being there.

The material is covered in a question and answer format, well validated and beloved by students, for rapid review and memorisation. This book is essential reading for any student (dental, medical, nursing, surgical assistant, operating department assistant, chiropody, podiatric) revising for exams, or for teachers who need a guide, or for anyone who works in theatre who needs to plug gaps in their knowledge. It is especially relevant for anyone contemplating the viva exams or the generic clinical skills section in exams of the various surgical colleges. Good luck.

Sam Andrews MA MS FRCS
Consultant General and Vascular Surgeon
Medway and Maidstone Hospitals, Kent, UK

Luke Cascarini BDS MB BCh FDSRCS MRCS
Specialist Registrar, Oral and Maxillofacial Surgery
South Thames region, Kent, UK

Acknowledgements

We would like to thank the following people for their help and guidance in the making of this book:

Alistair Challinor

Debbie Raher

David Lowe

Astrid Cunningham

Lizzie Baillie

Gill Bradham

Bryony Andrews

Nikki Bramhill

Dedication

To our children,

without whom it would have

been so much easier

Section 1

Aspects of pre-operative care

Chapter 1

Pre-operative investigations

1. Pre-admission clinic

What is the purpose of the pre-admission clinic (PAC)?

- To assess the patient's medical condition and optimise it pre-operatively if necessary.
- To check that the planned procedure is still appropriate and to continue the process of informed consent.
- To make arrangement for any special procedures or facilities which might be required, such as frozen section histopathology specimens or a booked ITU bed.
- To identify any appropriate investigations and ensure that any reports available have been seen and checked by the senior person responsible.

Who should be present at the PAC?

The PAC should be anaesthetic-led and provided by specialist nurses and person(s) from the admitting surgical team. Access to senior surgical advice should also be available for complex cases and those with significant comorbid conditions. Patients identified as high risk should be seen by the consultant anaesthetist.

Briefly outline the process of 'clerking a patient'

Clerking a surgical patient is an essential process of formally admitting the patient under a consultant's care. Patients can be 'pre-clerked' in the PAC, or clerked on admission.

Clerking a patient requires taking a full history, including details of the presenting symptoms, past medical history, family and social history, and drug and allergy history. The history should be completed by a full systematic enquiry of other relevant medical symptoms. The patient is then examined, with particular attention paid to the signs of the presenting condition and other systems that may affect the peri-operative management, e.g. cardiorespiratory system in patients undergoing general anaesthetic.

After formal clerking, appropriate investigations are arranged, the consent is checked, the drug chart is completed and any other arrangements, such as antibiotic prophylaxis, 'marking the patient', shaving or bowel preparation, are arranged.

2. Pre-operative haematology

What information does a pre-operative full blood count (FBC) provide?

A full blood count provides haemoglobin concentration, white cell count and platelet count. Haemoglobin concentration (12-16g/dl in male, 11-14g/dl in female), is a measure of the oxygen-carrying capacity of the blood. White cell count (5-10 x 10^9/l) is raised in the presence of infection. Platelet count (150-450 x 10^9/l) is one measure of blood clotting. A FBC may also provide details of red cell morphology (e.g. microcytosis in iron deficiency, macrocytosis in folate deficiency) and white cell differential (e.g. neutrophilia, leucopenia).

1.1.2

Which patients require a pre-operative FBC?

◆ All elective pre-operative patients over 60 years old, adult females or patients with a suspicion of anaemia, blood loss, haematological disease, cardiorespiratory conditions, sepsis or coagulation problems.

◆ All emergency pre-operative patients, especially those with abdominal conditions, malignancy, trauma and sepsis.

◆ All patients for surgery that could incur significant blood loss.

When should we ask for clotting studies?

Any patients on anticoagulants, with liver disease, or with a known clotting disorder should have pre-operative clotting studies. Clotting studies are important for patients having epidural anaesthesia (see section 2.6.1), as abnormal clotting can lead to spinal haematoma.

The prothrombin time (11-13 secs) measures the clotting factors of the extrinsic pathway. It is prolonged in patients on warfarin, and those with liver disease or disseminated intravascular coagulation (DIC).

The activated partial thromboplastin time (APTT) (<35 secs) measures the clotting factors of the intrinsic pathway. It is prolonged in heparin therapy, haemophilia and DIC. It used to be called the kaolin-cephalin clotting time (KCCT).

Why do some patients need a sickle test?

Patients of Afro-Caribbean origin may carry the gene for abnormal haemoglobin causing sickle cell disease. This may not be clinically obvious and can manifest itself at times of physical stress such as that caused by surgery. All patients of Afro-Caribbean origin should be pre-operatively tested.

3. Pre-operative biochemistry

When should the surgical team consider pre-operative urea and electrolyte (U & E) estimation?

Standard U & E estimation provides plasma concentrations of:

◆ Sodium (133-144mmol/l).
◆ Potassium (3.3-4.8mmol/l).
◆ Urea (2.5-6.5mmol/l).
◆ Creatinine (55-125μmol/l).

Pre-operative U & Es should be performed in all patients undergoing major surgery, and in all patients over 65 years.

Patients with concomitant cardiopulmonary disease, hepatic or renal disease, or metabolic or endocrine disorders may have deranged U & Es. In addition, pre-operative U & Es should be checked in all patients with a history of diarrhoea or vomiting, or with malnutrition, or those who are taking medications which might affect U & E concentrations, e.g. diuretics, steroids, cardiovascular medications, or who are on an intravenous infusion.

Which patients require pre-operative urinanalysis?

Urinanalysis testing provides evidence of the following substances in the urine: protein, blood, glucose, bilirubin, urobilinogen, ketones, nitrites, leucocytes, and urine pH and specific gravity. It does not provide exact urine concentrations, but does provide some quantitative information (negative, +, ++, +++, etc.).

Routine pre-operative urinanalysis should be performed on all emergency cases with abdominal or pelvic pain, in patients with abdominal or pelvic trauma and in diabetics.

A urine pregnancy test is performed in women of childbearing age with abdominal symptoms, or who require X-rays.

When is blood-glucose testing required pre-operatively?

The normal range for random blood glucose is 3-7mmol/l. It should be performed in all pre-operative patients with diabetes mellitus, malnutrition or obesity; patients presenting with abscesses, cellulitis or unusual infections; all patients over 60 years; and when glycosuria or ketonuria is present on urinanalysis.

What information is provided by liver function tests (LFTs)?

All pre-operative patients with upper abdominal pain, jaundice, malnutrition, known hepatic dysfunction, a history of alcohol abuse, or who are taking hepatically-metabolised medication should have pre-operative LFTs.

LFTs provide plasma concentrations of:

◆ Bilirubin (3-25μmol/l).
◆ Alkaline phosphatase (30-120iU/l).
◆ Alanine transaminase (ALT)/aspartate transaminase (AST) (10-60iU/l).
◆ Albumin (39-50g/l).
◆ Gamma-GT (10-80iU/l).

In addition, emergency pre-operative patients with abdominal pain should have amylase estimation.

4. Principles of pre-operative radiology

What information is required for referral for a radiology investigation?

Requesting an imaging investigation should be considered the same as a referral for any other specialist medical opinion. The best chance of getting the most from any investigation is to ensure the person doing the investigation is as fully informed as possible. Reasons for the request must be clear and a full medical and surgical history should be given. In complex cases, it is often best to go and talk to the radiologist.

1.1.4

What information should appear on an X-ray request form?

- Patient's name and address.
- Hospital ID number.
- Date of birth/age.
- Ward/department.
- Details of request, e.g. X-ray, ultrasound, CT, MRI.
- Area to be imaged, e.g. head, thorax, abdomen.
- Clinical details.
- Consultant's name.
- Relevant comorbidities, e.g. diabetic (metformin), renal failure.
- Mobility status (walking/wheelchair/trolley).
- Pregnancy status (date of last menstrual period) if relevent.
- Infection status, e.g. HIV, MRSA.
- Contrast allergies if known.
- Signature.
- Date.

What are the most common faults when using the radiology department?

- Repeating investigations which have already been done.
- Requesting investigations which will not change the patient's management.
- Failing to provide appropriate information to allow investigation to be properly interpreted.
- Over-investigation or unnecessary investigation.

5. Pre-operative X-rays

What pre-operative imaging may be required prior to surgery?

Pre-operative imaging may be done as part of the diagnostic investigation of the patient, e.g. barium enema examination for change in bowel habit, CT scan for investigation of internal bleeding following head injury. Pre-operative imaging is also used to provide a road map of the anatomy or pathology prior to surgical intervention, e.g. arteriography prior to vascular bypass surgery or CT staging prior to liver resection. It may also be done to investigate concomitant medical illness, prior to surgery or anaesthesia, e.g. pre-operative chest X-ray (see below) or cervical spine X-ray for patients with arthritis. It is essential that all pre-operative radiology imaging is sent to theatre with the patient.

Which patients should get a pre-operative chest X-ray?

All elective pre-operative patients over 60 years old, patients with cervical, thoracic or abdominal trauma, patients with previous or concurrent cardiorespiratory disease, patients with malignancy or goitre, and patients with previous tuberculosis or close TB contacts.

How are X-ray images viewed in the operating theatre?

Conventional X-ray films are viewed on an X-ray box, hung in the operating theatre, where they can be easily seen from where the surgeon is standing. Computer-generated images can be viewed on a computer screen in the theatre.

When may intra-operative radiology be required?

Intra-operative imaging is performed as an adjunct to surgery, to guide surgery, or to make on-table diagnosis, e.g. real time, image-intensifier images in orthopaedic surgery, to guide the position of orthopaedic prostheses, or intra-operative cholangiography during open or laparoscopic cholecystectomy to diagnose bile duct stones.

6. Problems with pre-operative radiology

What are the general rules governing the use of ionising radiation?

The use of ionising radiation must be justified in terms of clear benefits to the patient, which should outweigh the radiation risks. Statutory regulations require all radiologists and radiographers to reduce unnecessary exposure of patients to radiation.

When is the foetus most sensitive to ionising radiation?

Any exposure of the foetus to radiation should be avoided where possible; however, the developing foetus is particularly sensitive to the effects of radiation during the period of organogenesis which is 2-9 weeks after conception.

Why are radiologists interested in the patient's allergies?

Contrast reactions to intravenous reagents can occasionally occur. Death from anaphylactic shock occurs in about 1 in 40,000 cases. Other possible sequelae include hives and pulmonary oedema. A history of atopy or allergy to iodine or seafood is especially important. Premedication with corticosteroids or the use of newer non-iodine-based contrast agents may be indicated.

Why are radiologists interested in renal impairment and diabetes?

Intravascular contrast studies with iodinated materials can lead to acute alteration of renal function. This has the potential to precipitate lactic acidosis in patients receiving metformin therapy. Metformin should be discontinued at the time of examination and for at least 48 hours after examination or until normal renal function is confirmed. It is imperative that the radiology department know of any patients receiving metformin therapy in advance of these investigations.

7. Other pre-operative investigations

Which patients require pre-operative electrocardiography (ECG)?

A 12-lead resting ECG is a useful test for detecting abnormalities of rate, rhythm, myocardial perfusion or previous infarction. However, it may still be normal in the presence of extensive coronary artery disease.

It should be performed pre-operatively in all patients over 60; patients undergoing cardiac, vascular or renal surgery; patients with hypertension, cardiovascular disease and taking cardiac medications; and patients with an irregular or abnormal pulse.

What other cardiac investigations might be considered?

Patients who have had a recent myocardial infarction should, if possible, be deferred until six months after the event. Patients with pre-operative cardiac symptoms (see section 1.2.5), or for major thoracic or vascular surgery might benefit from echocardiography or even coronary angiography, so any occult coronary stenoses can be considered for angioplasty, before major surgery is considered. Patients with cardiac arrhythmias should have a 24-hour cardiac monitor, a cardiology opinion and pre-operative correction if feasible. Patients with pacemakers should have a pre-operative pacemaker check.

What are respiratory function tests?

Respiratory function tests are performed to ascertain the extent of pre-operative respiratory disease, to predict postoperative function and complications, and to act as a baseline prior to thoracic surgery. They include blood gas analysis and spirometric studies. Spirometry measures the volume of air forced out in the first second of expiration (FEV1) and the total amount forced out (FVC), and thus the FEV1/FVC ratio can be derived (see section 1.2.3).

Why might the anaesthetist be interested in pre-operative arterial blood gas analysis?

Arterial blood gases provide:

- pO_2 (10-14kPa, 75-100mmHg).
- pCO_2 (4-6kPa, 35-42mmHg).
- pH (7.35-7.45).
- HCO_3^- (23-33mmol/l).
- Lactate (0.7-2.1mmol/l).

In addition, some blood gas machines provide information on oxygen saturation, base excess, haemoglobin concentration, and urea and electrolyte concentrations.

Blood gas analysis provides information on oxygenation, CO_2 excretion and acid base balance. It is a measure of respiratory, renal and cardiovascular function. It is used as a baseline prior to major surgery, to identify occult respiratory failure and to elucidate other metabolic disturbances.

Chapter 2

Management of concomitant medical conditions

1. General management of associated medical conditions

What patient groups are considered high risk for surgery?

- Extremes of age:
  - elderly;
  - infants;
  - neonates.
- Obese patients (body mass index >30).
- Smokers.
- Those with pre-existing diseases especially:
  - cardiorespiratory problems;
  - malignancy;
  - hypertension;
  - diabetes;
  - liver failure;
  - renal diseases;
  - rheumatoid diseases.
- Patients on multiple medications.
- Immunosuppressed patients.
- Patients with coagulopathies.
- Pregnant patients.
- Malnourished patients.

What special measures can be performed to reduce peri-operative risk?

General measures:

◆ Perform high risk operations at the beginning of the list to maximise 'daylight hours' recovery time and reduce starvation time.
◆ Operate early in the week if possible (often less staff around at weekends).
◆ Ensure consultant is informed.
◆ Ensure senior surgeon and anaesthetist are available.
◆ Notify theatres (place details on printed operating list).

Specific measures depend upon the condition - see the following sections.

2. Elderly patients

Why are elderly patients at increased risk of surgery?

Although biological age is more important than chronological age, generally elderly people have less cardiorespiratory reserve and more concurrent illnesses, they are more likely to be on multiple medications and have mobility problems. As a result, they often take longer to recover after operations and spend longer in hospital, which may be one of the reasons why they also succumb to more postoperative infections. They are more prone to stroke, delirium, deep venous thrombosis and fluid overload.

Who can help with the discharge of elderly patients and how?

◆ Discharge planning should begin at pre-assessment or on admission.
◆ An occupational therapy (OT) assessment can be arranged pre-operatively.
◆ Physiotherapy need not be reserved for postoperative patients; by then it may be too late. Pre-operative breathing and mobility exercises speed recovery.

- Pre-operative nutritional status needs dietician assessment and optimisation.
- Social workers and community support teams are essential to help elderly patients return to their pre-operative lifestyle. This requires early planning and close liaison between the hospital and community teams.

3. Respiratory diseases

Why are pre-operative respiratory conditions important?

Anaesthesia and surgery have deleterious effects on respiratory function. Patients with pre-existing respiratory disease are much more likely to have postoperative respiratory problems. In addition, respiratory diseases have effects on other systems; most importantly, the cardiovascular system, increasing the likelihood of cardiovascular complications. For example, if the lungs are working sub-optimally and the arterial oxygen saturation is low, this may cause an increase in cardiac output which may precipitate an ischaemic cardiac event.

If the vital capacity is less than three times tidal volume then respiratory insufficiency is very likely after a laparotomy or thoracotomy, because the pain and muscle cutting cause the vital capacity to be reduced by about two thirds. By testing pulmonary function pre-operatively this can be pre-empted so it may be possible, either through employing minimally invasive surgical techniques or epidural anaesthesia, to prevent respiratory complications.

If pulmonary function tests show there is pre-existing bronchospasm, there is an increased risk of sputum retention and pneumonia. This risk can be minimised by optimising medical therapy pre-operatively. This usually involves the use of bronchodilators such as salbutamol.

Patients with pre-existing restrictive lung disease are at risk of postoperative respiratory failure through fatigue. By being aware of this risk, special measures can be employed to reduce this risk, by using minimally invasive techniques if possible.

How would you assess a patient who is asthmatic?

History: duration of condition, effects on normal life, previous worst severity, any episodes of hospital attendance, admission, ITU, intubation, and current and previous medication, especially oral steroids. Precipitating factors: seasonal, exercise, illness-related. Normal peak expiratory flow rate (PEFR) and smoking history are also important.

Examination:

◆ **Look** - for dyspnoea, tachypnoea.
◆ **Listen** - for wheezes, pneumothorax.
◆ **Feel** - for equal expansion, tactile vocal fremitis.

Investigations:

◆ PEFR is essential.
◆ Pulmonary function tests are highly desirable in all, but very well controlled, mild asthmatics.
◆ Chest X-ray and blood gas analysis in moderate and severe cases.

Outline the differences between obstructive and restrictive pulmonary disease

In obstructive disease the patient's major problem is the inability to move air in and out, although the actual total amount of air moved can also be reduced. The ratio between amount forced out in the first second (FEV1) and total amount forced out (FVC) is reduced due to an obstruction of the airways, e.g. asthma, tumours, chronic obstructive pulmonary disease (COPD).

In restrictive disease the volumes of inspired and expired air are reduced but the rate of flow is not altered much or may be increased. Thus, the ratio between amount expired in the first second and total amount is high (FEV1/FVC approximately 90%), e.g. chest wall problems, fibrosis, pulmonary oedema and post-lung surgery.

4. Smoking

How does smoking increase the risks of surgery?

Carbon monoxide reduces oxygen delivery to tissues. Nicotine increases heart rate and can cause peripheral vasoconstriction. Bronchociliary function is impaired. Long-term smoking further impairs pulmonary function usually causing obstructive-type respiratory symptoms. Smoking also impairs the immune system and causes atherosclerosis, increasing ischaemic heart disease and peripheral vascular disease.

How can the risks be reduced?

Smoking cessation helps. Carbon monoxide and nicotine levels return to normal within 12-24 hours. Ciliary function starts to improve after 2-3 days. After three months of abstention, lung function returns to normal. Pre-operative optimisation for smokers also includes physiotherapy, oxygen and bronchodilator therapy.

How can the surgical team help patients to stop smoking pre-operatively?

There is evidence that medical professionals can have a significant impact on patients' smoking behaviour. Advice and encouragement can be combined with written information and direction towards specialist clinics and help groups. Nicotine supplements can help the patient overcome the pharmacological addiction to nicotine. These are taken in many ways including chewing gum, nasal inhalant, sub-lingual tablets and by drawing on a plastic 'cigarette'. Other drugs which can help are Zyban™ (bupropion hydrochloride) and Champix™ (varenicline). Zyban™ is a weak inhibitor of neuronal uptake of dopamine, serotonin and noradrenaline and is thought to reduce the craving for nicotine. Champix™ binds to nicotine receptors in the brain and reduces the nicotine withdrawal symptoms, and also reduces the satisfaction a smoker gets from a cigarette.

Non-pharmaceutical means to quit smoking include hypnotism and cognitive behavioural therapy.

5. Cardiac disease

What are the important cardiac risk factors?

Important cardiac risk factors are:

- Signs of cardiac failure.
- Myocardial infarction in the last six months.
- More than five premature ventricular beats per minute.
- Arrhythmias.
- Hypertension.
- Age over 70.
- Emergency surgery.
- Vascular, thoracic or abdominal surgery.
- Aortic stenosis.
- Poor general physical condition.

How can cardiac function be assessed before surgery?

- History - exercise tolerance, paroxysmal nocturnal dyspnoea, orthopnoea, ankle swelling, chest pain.
- Examination - rate, rhythm, oedema, jugular venous pressure.
- Investigations - electrocardiogram, echocardiography, exercise tolerance test (treadmill), angiography, thallium scan.

What classification systems do you know for patients with heart disease?

The two most common systems are:

The New York Heart Association classification of patients with heart disease
Class 1 - Asymptomatic.
Class 2 - Symptoms with ordinary activity, but comfortable at rest.

Class 3 - Symptoms with minimal activity, but comfortable at rest.
Class 4 - Symptoms at rest.

New York Heart Association risk of peri-operative MI
Class 1 - Angina with strenuous exercise.
Class 2 - Angina with moderate exercise.
Class 3 - Angina after climbing one flight of stairs.
Class 4 - Angina with any exercise.

How does a general anaesthetic increase the risk of an acute coronary event?

Sudden increases in myocardial oxygen demand, such as an increase in heart rate or blood pressure, or reductions in oxygen supply (hypoxaemia, hypotension or anaemia) can precipitate myocardial infarction in patients with ischaemic heart disease.

6. Hypertension

Which organs are particularly damaged by hypertension?

Longstanding hypertension will cause ventricular hypertrophy and congestive cardiac failure. The other organs liable to injury are the so called end organs. These are the brain, the kidneys, and the eyes.

What are the secondary causes of hypertension?

Ninety-five percent of hypertensive patients have essential or primary hypertension where the cause is unknown.

Secondary hypertension is caused by:

◆ Renal disease - renal artery stenosis, congenital polycystic kidneys, chronic glomerulonephritis.
◆ Endocrine disease - Cushing's, Conn's, phaeochromocytoma, acromegaly, hyperparathyroidism.

- Neurogenic causes - psychogenic, raised intracranial pressure, spinal cord transection, polyneuritis.
- Others - coarctation of the aorta, steroids and pregnancy.

Why is it important to control hypertension pre-operatively?

Hypertension is a major risk factor for myocardial infarction, renal failure, left ventricular failure and strokes. This is true whether the patient is having surgery or not; surgery is an additional risk factor.

How is hypertension managed?

A patient with raised blood pressure should be fully assessed through history, examination and investigations. The aims of this assessment should be to see if the hypertension is a one-off response to a perceived threatening situation (in hospital this is commonly called white coat hypertension) or if it is a longstanding problem. Once it has been determined that this is not white coat hypertension, then it is necessary to assess if it is 'essential' or 'secondary' hypertension. It is also important to assess what damage has been done by the hypertension.

In a hospital setting if a patient's blood pressure is high and they are due to have an operation imminently the options are limited. The operation can be cancelled and the patient can be seen by their general practitioner for management, or the surgery can proceed with or without medication given pre-operatively to reduce the blood pressure. Generally speaking, mild to moderate hypertension (diastolic below 110mm Hg) does not warrant cancellation of surgery but the patient may benefit from a beta-blocker pre-operatively. Postoperatively, they should be advised to see their general practitioner for further management. If the blood pressure is any higher then it is usually an unnecessary risk to proceed with elective surgery.

Mild to moderate essential hypertension can be controlled with weight loss, regular exercise and cutting down on alcohol and salt consumption. However, these are often unrealistic goals and the hypertension is more often controlled with diuretics, beta-blockers, ACE inhibitors or calcium channel blockers. Refractory hypertension is best managed by a specialist.

Hypertensive patients should receive their normal antihypertensive medication pre-operatively to prevent rebound hypertension in the postoperative period.

7. Obesity

What is body mass index (BMI) and how is it calculated?

BMI is weight / height ^{2}, weight in kilograms and height in metres. The ideal is 20-25.

How does obesity increase the surgical complication rate?

Complications directly related to obesity can be divided into pre-operative, peri-operative and postoperative.

Pre-operatively, obese patients are more difficult to examine due to the layer of adipose tissue covering the organs. For example, abdominal tenderness may be less marked or a parotid lump may be less distinct. This can lead to delayed or inaccurate diagnosis. Venous access and fine needle aspiration cytology is more difficult which can make sampling difficult or inaccurate and lead to under-investigation. Obese individuals have a higher prevalence of pre-existing medical diseases such as diabetes, osteoarthritis, reflux gastritis, hypertension, heart failure and deep vein thrombosis, all of which increase the risks of complications from surgery.

Peri-operatively, obesity makes surgery more technically challenging which may result in procedures taking longer and involve larger incisions to gain adequate access. Technical aspects, such as moving the anaesthetised patient, are more complex and may lead to iatrogenic complications such as nerve injury. Anaesthetic problems can result from abnormal pharmacokinetics due to fat absorption and release, as well as the pre-existing medical problems. Mask ventilation and intubation are more difficult and airway obstruction is also a potential problem. Increased abdominal fat leads to hiatus hernia and increases the risk of aspiration. Spinal anaesthesia and nerve blocks are also more of a problem. Anaesthetic monitoring may be more difficult; blood pressure measurements may be inaccurate and especially large blood pressure cuffs may be required.

Postoperatively, obese patients are more likely to suffer wound complications, such as haematoma, infection and dehiscence due to difficulty in achieving adequate wound closure (fat cannot be properly sutured but its weight pulls the fascial layers apart). They are also more likely to suffer incisional herniation, deep venous thrombosis, stroke and myocardial infarction.

8. Diabetes

Why is it important to maintain control of blood sugar peri-operatively?

High levels of blood glucose leads to increased risk of infection, poor wound healing, osmotic diuresis and dehydration. The insulin deficiency may lead to keto-acidosis and protein catabolism.

How should a non-insulin-dependent diabetic be managed for surgery?

Non-insulin-dependent diabetics are at risk of hypoglycaemia, which if unnoticed, could lead to severe brain injury, coma and death. They should:

◆ Be first on the list.
◆ Stop oral hypoglycaemic drugs on the day of surgery.
◆ Have an intravenous cannula with slow infusion, about 100ml per hour of 5% dextrose/saline mixture.
◆ Have regular blood sugar tests and start a sliding scale if necessary.
◆ Restart their medications as soon as possible after surgery when they can eat.

Different establishments may have different local protocols. If in doubt discuss with the anaesthetist first.

How should insulin-dependent diabetics be managed?

◆　Admit on the day before operation.
◆　Be first on the list.
◆　Stop long-acting insulin the night before operation.
◆　Check electrolytes on the morning of surgery.
◆　Do not give the normal morning dose - start a sliding scale.
◆　When the patient can eat again return to the normal insulin regimen.

What is meant by a sliding scale insulin regimen?

A sliding scale is an infusion of insulin and glucose that varies the amount given according to the blood glucose level. Five percent dextrose is administered intravenously at 100ml per hour, with 50 units short-acting insulin in 50ml normal saline via an infusion pump given according to the regimen below. Patients must be closely monitored and have regular blood glucose tests.

A normal regimen is shown in Table 1 (this is only a guide).

Table 1. Sliding scale insulin regimen.

Glucose	Insulin units/hour
<2	Give 50% glucose intravenously and arrange medical assistance
2-5	0
5-10	1
10-15	2
15-20	3
>20	6 and arrange medical assistance

What drugs can interfere with blood sugar control?

The most common drugs to cause hyperglycaemia are corticosteroids. Thiazide diuretics may also precipitate hyperglycaemia in a minority of patients.

Blood glucose can be lowered by alcohol and phenytoin. It is also wise to use beta-blockers cautiously in diabetic patients, as they may mask the symptoms of hypoglycaemia.

9. Pregnancy

What are the principles of surgical management of the pregnant patient?

Non-emergency surgery should be avoided to protect the foetus. The second trimester is the safest time to operate. Manipulation of the uterus should be avoided to prevent premature labour.

There is a significant risk of aspiration of gastric contents during induction of anaesthesia and the anaesthetist will probably give an antacid pre-operatively and use cricoid pressure with rapid sequence intubation to minimise this risk (see section 1.3.10).

How does pregnancy alter patient positioning on the operating table?

It is usually preferable to avoid the supine position as in this position the gravid uterus may compress the inferior vena cava and the aorta. Caval compression causes reduction in venous return to the heart which manifests as hypotension, tachycardia, pallor, sweating, nausea and vomiting, much like shock. Compression of the aorta causes a decrease in uterine blood flow and may lead to foetal distress.

1.2.9

What are the most common operations in pregnancy other than delivering the foetus?

The most common surgical problems requiring operation in pregnancy are appendicitis, torsion or rupture of ovarian cysts, cholecystitis and trauma.

What special considerations should be made with regard to drugs in pregnancy?

The prescriber must always consider the effects of the drug on both mother and foetus. For many drugs there is insufficient evidence whether it is truly safe or not, so avoid prescribing unless there is good reason to do so and always check in a formulary if the drug is contraindicated in pregnancy. Generally the earlier in pregnancy the drug is given the greater the risk of teratogenesis.

10. Liver disease

Why are patients with liver disease especially at risk during surgical procedures?

Excessive bleeding is a major risk due to reduced absorption of vitamin K, leading to reduced synthesis of clotting factors II, VII, IX and X, causing increased prothrombin time. Portal hypertension causing hypersplenism may also lead to thrombocytopenia and reduced platelet activity.

Hypoalbuminaemia leading to fluid overload is common in jaundiced patients. This may lead to pulmonary or peripheral oedema, or ascites. Hypoalbuminaemic patients also have poor wound healing.

The risk of infection is increased as the high levels of bilirubin suppress the immune system. Renal failure may also occur due to absorption of endotoxin from the gut leading to hepatorenal syndrome. Depleted glycogen stores may precipitate hypoglycaemia.

1.2.10

Many drugs, including anaesthetic agents, are metabolised by the liver, so they may have a prolonged duration. Low serum albumin affects the action of drugs with high protein binding.

What special measures do patients with jaundice require?

Surgery should be avoided in jaundiced patients if possible. If the jaundice can be relieved pre-operatively, e.g. by endoscopic sphincterotomy or percutaneous transhepatic drainage, this should be considered.

If surgery is essential, pre-operative vitamin K can be given, and fresh frozen plasma administered peri-operatively to facilitate clotting. Patients must be well hydrated pre-operatively and a loop or osmotic diuretic is given on induction to maximise renal output. Hepatorenal syndrome may also be prevented by pre-operative administration of lactulose or bile salts.

Systemic, broad-spectrum antibiotics are given on induction as infection prophylaxis.

11. Thyroid disease

What do you look for specifically when examining a pre-operative patient with goitre?

- ◆ Look for signs of hyper- or hypothyroidism.
- ◆ Look for signs that the goitre is causing partial or imminent airway obstruction, especially if extending retrosternally.
- ◆ Look for distended veins in the neck suggesting venous obstruction.
- ◆ The vocal cords should also be examined.

What investigations would you request?

- ◆ Initial investigations for goitre are ultrasound with fine needle aspiration if there are cysts or nodules.

◆   Blood tests include thyroid function, thyroid antibodies, full blood count, calcium and electrolytes.

◆   Ultrasound can show retrosternal extension and the effect of neck extension, but CT or MRI is required to show full retrosternal extent and tracheal compromise.

◆   Nuclear medicine is reserved for selected cases on the request of a specialist.

What is the pre-operative preparation for a hyperthyroid patient?

Hyperthyroid patients must be rendered euthyroid prior to surgery whenever possible. This is because surgery in the hyperthyroid patient is fraught with complications mainly due to the hyperdynamic state of the circulation which can lead to atrial fibrillation, arrhythmias and ischaemic cardiac events. Furthermore, a thyroid storm may be precipitated by the stress of the surgery which may lead to extreme tachycardia, hyperthermia and possibly hypotension; it can be mistaken for malignant hyperpyrexia. Also, thyroid surgery itself is more complicated in the hyperthyroid state as the thyroid gland is more swollen and vascular, and likely to bleed excessively, be more difficult to remove and there is an increased chance of nerve injury.

The patient may be rendered euthyroid with carbimazole or propyl thiouracil or Lugol's iodine. Beta-blockers, such as propranolol, can also help prevent the cardiovascular problems.

12. Rheumatoid disease

Why is rheumatoid disease of concern to the surgical team?

The surgeon may be operating on a rheumatoid patient for reasons directly relating to their disease, such as joint replacement, or because a patient with rheumatoid disease may be having an operation for an unrelated condition.

Describe its effects on the major body systems

Rheumatoid disease is a multi-system autoimmune disorder. Its effects can be grouped into those directly related to the disease itself and those related to the treatments given. The joint destruction is important as patients must be moved and positioned with extreme care; they are at risk of cervical spine instability (especially atlanto-axial subluxation) and also partly because of this and disease in the temporomandibular joint, laryngoscopy for intubation is often difficult. Intubation can also be made difficult by rheumatoid disease of the crico-arytenoid joints. The disease may cause alveolitis and pulmonary fibrosis as well as pleuritis and pleural effusions. The heart can be affected, including pericarditis, valve disorders and conduction abnormalities. Patients may also have anaemia of chronic disease and may be immunocompromised. The kidneys can be affected by non-steroidal anti-inflammatory drugs (NSAID), gold and penicillamine, as well as secondary to amyloid deposition. The treatments may also be immunosuppressant or, in the case of NSAIDs, cause gastric bleeding.

What investigations would be helpful?

Patients should have a chest X-ray, pulmonary function tests, echocardiography, a full blood work-up and will often need flexion-extension X-rays of their neck, especially if they have a reduced range of movement or neck pain - discuss with the anaesthetist first.

13. Renal disease

How would you assess pre-operative renal function?

Renal function can be assessed in terms of glomerular and tubular function.

The glomerulus acts as a pressure filter producing an ultrafiltrate of plasma. The glomerular filtration rate (GFR) is a measure of glomerular function and depends upon body size, sex, age, renal blood supply and degree of nephron destruction through renal disease. The GFR is

1.2.13

estimated by measuring the creatinine clearance. This is calculated from the creatinine content of a 24-hour urine collection and the plasma creatinine concentration during this period.

The serum concentrations of creatinine and urea (renal function tests) are much more convenient measures, but are less sensitive because the GFR must fall to about half its normal level before there is a significant rise in serum creatinine concentration. Serum urea level is also a poor indication of renal function as dietary protein will affect serum urea concentration, as can gastrointestinal bleeding. However, serum urea and creatinine levels and their ratios are useful in the investigation of renal dysfunction.

The renal tubules are responsible for reabsorption of water, glucose and amino acids. There are no simple tests which can measure tubular function quantitatively. However, a comparison of urine and serum osmolality measurements will show if a patient can concentrate their urine normally.

How would you manage a patient with end-stage renal failure who requires elective surgery?

It is essential that the renal team are informed and involved in the perioperative care of these patients. If it is a quick procedure requiring little in-patient time it may be possible to fit the operation in between dialysis sessions. Ideally, surgery should be deferred until 24 hours after dialysis so that the fluid shifts have settled. More prolonged stay will require arrangements to be made for dialysis. When managing these patients it is important to be aware that they are immunocompromised, usually anaemic, easily fluid overloaded and have electrolyte abnormalities, especially hypercalcaemia, hyponatraemia, acidosis and hyperkalaemia. Renal physicians are exceedingly proficient at managing these patients, most surgeons are not; it is hard to justify not seeking their help.

1.2.14

14. Immunosuppressed patients

What types of immunocompromise might be encountered in surgical practice?

Congenital:

◆ Non-specific immunosuppression, e.g. chronic granulomatous disease leads to recurrent abscesses; complement deficiency is rare and may lead to recurrent bacterial infection.
◆ Primary antibody deficiencies such as X-linked agammaglobulinaemia.
◆ T-cell deficiencies such as Di-George syndrome.

Acquired (most common):

◆ Alcohol excess.
◆ Smoking.
◆ IV drug abuse.
◆ Poverty.
◆ Old age.
◆ Chronic illness (rheumatoid arthritis, renal and liver diseases, diabetes).
◆ Drugs, including steroids and immunosuppressants.
◆ Haematological cancer and its treatment.
◆ HIV.

What special precautions should you take?

Precautions to protect patients include liaison with appropriate specialists, use of all appropriate measures to optimise patients' general physical condition and specifically their immunological status, and steps taken to minimise risk of infection (see section 1.3.6).

Precautions are also taken to protect hospital staff in cases where a patient may present an infection risk, although nowadays most hospitals accept that universal precautions should be adequate (see section 1.4.7).

What features of a patient's history might alert you to the possibility of as yet undiagnosed immunocompromise?

Patients who present with unusually severe infection, infection at unusual sites, recurrent infection or unusual pathogens should lead to investigations for immunosuppression.

15. Pre-operative management of patients taking steroids

Which patients might need pre-operative steroid cover?

Patients who have been on long-term steroid therapy within the last year may develop suppression of the hypothalamus-pituitary-adrenal axis (HPA) and are, therefore, at risk of developing acute peri-operative adrenal insufficiency. There is inadequate evidence to predict exactly what dose of steroids and for how long they must be taken to cause this effect. However, since peri-operative steroid cover has few side effects and acute adrenal insufficiency can lead to death, most experts advocate supplemental steroids be given if there is any doubt about the patient's HPA.

Outline the recommended steroid cover for minor and major procedures

The doses of supplemental steroids should take into account the duration of therapy, the dose taken pre-operatively and the degree of surgical stress. However, there is little hard evidence for the safest regimen. The case should be discussed with the anaesthetist or the endocrinologist. One simple regimen advocates 25mg of hydrocortisone intravenously for minor surgery and for major surgery 25mg hydrocortisone intra-operatively followed by 100mg infused over 24 hours postoperatively.

What is the steroid cover aiming to prevent?

Acute peri-operative adrenal insufficiency or an Addisonian crisis. This may present with rigidity, vomiting, collapse and refractory hypotension. It may be mistaken for an acute abdominal emergency. There will be low serum cortisol levels and there may also be hyponatraemia and hyperkalaemia.

How is it managed?

Urgent intravenous hydrocortisone, fluid replacement, close monitoring and correction of electrolyte abnormalities including glucose.

16. Pre-operative management of patients taking anticoagulants

What are the common anticoagulants patients might be taking pre-operatively?

1.2.16

◆ Those that work to block Vitamin K synthesis which are derived from 4-hydroxycoumarin; the most well known is warfarin. This is one of the most common problematic drugs as it interacts with many other drugs which can cause inadvertent and dangerous prolongation of prothrombin time. Patients taking warfarin should stop taking it five days prior to surgery and have their clotting checked pre-operatively. Patients who need ongoing anticoagulation, e.g. those with artificial heart valves should be converted to heparin anticoagulation. In the emergency situation warfarin anticoagulation can be reversed with fresh frozen plasma, or vitamin K.

◆ Those that potentiate the activity of antithrombin III - the heparins which are classified as unfractionated and low molecular weight.

◆ Antiplatelet drugs - clopidogrel and aspirin.

What effects does aspirin have on the blood?

Aspirin inhibits platelet activity by irreversibly blocking cyclo-oxygenase, preventing platelet activation and aggregation, and hence blood clotting.

Some surgery is best postponed until after the effects of the aspirin have worn off, as the additional bleeding may be difficult to control, e.g. following transurethral resection of the prostate, or may cause an unacceptable degree of bruising and potential infections, e.g. plastic surgical facelifts, or free flaps. Aspirin can also cause gastric bleeding and perforation.

Aspirin needs to be stopped for at least seven days pre-operatively for there to be any difference, as this is the approximate half-life of platelets.

What is thrombophilia and why is this important?

Thrombophilia is the name given to a group of conditions where there is an increased propensity for blood clotting. The commonest cause of acquired thrombophilia is malignancy. Congenital thrombophilias include protein S and protein C deficiency, lupus anticoagulant and factor V Leiden, antithrombin (formerly antithrombin III) deficiency, prothrombin 20210 and dysfibrinogenaemia.

Patients with thrombophilia are more prone to deep vein thrombosis, and may be taking anticoagulants.

17. Pre-operative management of other medications

How does the oral contraceptive pill increase the risk of surgical complications?

The combined oestrogen and progesterone contraceptive pill increases the risk of postoperative deep vein thrombosis. This is due to reducing the activity of antithrombin III.

1.2.17

What potential problems can arise with cardiac medications?

- Digoxin can cause toxicity, including nausea, vomiting, arrhythmias and heart block. It is important to avoid digitalis toxicity which is more likely in the elderly and in hypokaleamia, hypomagnesaemia and hypercalcaemia. If in doubt check the plasma levels.
- Calcium channel blocker, Verapamil, can cause heart block, bradycardia and hypotension and should not be used with beta-blockers. Nifedipine causes reflex tachycardia and is often used with a beta-blocker.
- Thiazide and loop diuretics can cause hypokaleamia and hypotension.
- Furosemide can cause hyperglycaemia. If a patient is hypovolaemic it is often useful to stop their diuretic whilst they are being rehydrated.
- Potassium-sparing diuretics can cause hyperkalaemia.
- ACE inhibitors can cause hyperkalaemia and hypotension as well as dry cough and oedema. Some anaesthetists prefer to stop ACE inhibitors prior to surgery due to the labile blood pressure they can cause.
- Beta-blockers cause bradycardia and hypotension and may mask the normal reaction to hypovolaemia.

What potential problems can arise with inhalers?

Salbutamol can cause tachycardia and hypokaleamia. Most patients are advised to use their inhalers as usual before surgery and anaesthesia.

Which medications should be stopped on the day of surgery?

- Diabetic medications (see section 1.2.8).
- Anticoagulants (see section 1.2.16).
- Some cardiac medications (see above).
- Other medications can be continued up to and including the day of surgery. Monoamine oxidase inhibitors can interact with many anaesthetic agents (particularly pethidine), but this does not usually mean they need to be stopped; it is usually sufficient for the anaesthetist to be aware so that interactions can be avoided.

Chapter 3

Preparation for theatre

1. Assessment of fitness for surgery

Do you know any risk assessment scoring systems?

The best known is the American Society of Anesthesiologists (ASA) physical status classification (see below). The POSSUM (Physiologic and Operative Severity Score for the enUmeration of Mortality and Morbidity) has 12 physiological results and allows the prediction of morbidity and mortality. It is used for comparing techniques and centres for elective surgery.

The Acute Physiology And Chronic Health Evaluation (APACHE) also has 12 physiological variables and can be used to predict outcome and appraise treatment methods; it is most useful in emergency surgery.

Describe the ASA system

- ◆ Class 1 - Healthy, no medical problems.
- ◆ Class 2 - Mild systemic disease.
- ◆ Class 3 - Severe systemic disease but not incapacitation.
- ◆ Class 4 - Severe systemic disease that is a constant threat to life.

◆ Class 5 - Moribund, not expected to live for more than 24 hours, irrespective of operation.

E is added to the number to represent emergency surgery.

For example, a patient for a knee replacement with unstable angina would be class 4, a well-controlled asthmatic with appendicitis would be class 2E.

Explain how risk scoring systems work and how they help the surgical team

Risk scoring systems use variables such as age and physiological measurements to predict morbidity and mortality. These statistics can be used in two ways. They can in certain cases be used to individually calculate the risk of morbidity and mortality for individual patients. However, by far the most common and accurate use is for epidemiological research purposes. They enable surgeons to compare their results with other surgeons and take into account factors which are beyond the control of the surgeon, such as pre-existing illness.

2. Optimisation of pre-operative nutritional status

How and why do we assess the nutritional status of patients pre-operatively?

1.3.2

Malnutrition is very common in pre-operative patients, and malnourished patients have higher morbidity and mortality rates.

Causes of pre-operative malnutrition include:

◆ An inability to eat, e.g. gastrointestinal obstruction or previous stroke.
◆ A catabolic state, e.g. weight loss due to malignancy.
◆ Social factors, e.g. elderly patient incapable of cooking and shopping due to poor support.

Nutritional state can be assessed by history (e.g. poor diet, weight loss), examination (e.g. cachexia, muscle weakness, peripheral oedema) and various physical or biochemical parameters:

Physical:

◆ Body mass index measurement.
◆ Triceps skin fold thickness.
◆ Hand grip strength.

Biochemical:

◆ Serum albumin estimation.
◆ Transferrin levels.
◆ Haemoglobin level.

Malnourished patients are best treated by pre-operative nutritional optimisation.

What techniques can be used to improve a patient's nutritional status?

Pre-operative feeding can be performed prior to elective non-urgent surgery to improve nutritional status prior to surgery. Enteral feeding includes dietary supplementation or nasogastric or nasojejunal tube feeding. Parenteral feed is administered intravenously.

For urgent or emergency surgery, peri- or postoperative feeding is required (see section 3.10.9).

Malnourished patients may have abnormal clotting, which will need to be corrected pre-operatively, and poor wound healing, so immaculate surgical technique is required. Stitches may need to be left in longer to give healing wounds more strength, and prophylactic antibiotics may be indicated.

3. Surgical marking

Why are patients 'marked'?

The process of marking a patient is part of a multi-stage process designed to prevent errors. An indelible marking pen is used to place a mark in the vicinity of the proposed incision. This helps to reduce the risk of performing the wrong operation, getting the wrong patient, or operating on the wrong side. So, if a patient is having a left-sided operation of any kind the patient should be marked on the left side.

Marking is also used to identify the exact site of the incision in situations where this may not be apparent, for example, the exact position of abdominal hernias is not always apparent when the patient is in the supine position, or the position of varicose veins may not be obvious with the patient supine with head down tilt.

Who should do the 'marking'?

Marking should follow the same rules as gaining consent, that is it should ideally be done by the operating surgeon or at least a member of the team who might be doing the operation. In practice, marking is often done by junior members of the team. It should always be checked by the operating surgeon.

What are the dangers of 'marking' patients?

Marking can be rubbed off, if performed too long before the proposed surgery. Some skin preparation will wash away non-indelible marks. Incisions through marks can cause skin tattooing. Marking can be transferred if marked skin is touched against non-marked skin whilst the mark is not dry. This is a particular hazard in lower limb surgery when the mark is placed on the medial side of the limb.

4. Principles of surgical prophylaxis

What are the principles of prophylaxis in relation to surgery?

Prophylactic measures are designed to minimise complications in surgery. To be effective the measure must be present throughout the time of risk. For example, with prophylactic antibiotics the drug must be at effective serum concentrations throughout the operation and be a bactericidal type. The measure must be proven to work and be of reasonably low risk itself.

In general, prophylaxis is used in two circumstances: firstly, when the risk is common and the potential risk of the prophylaxis is low such as prophylactic antibiotics for bowel surgery; secondly, where the risk is rare but the consequences are horrendous and the prophylaxis is reasonably safe, for example, prophylactic antibiotics for dental procedures in patients with prosthetic heart valves where, although bacterial endocarditis is rare, there is a very high mortality rate.

What are the risks against which surgeons regularly use prophylactic measures?

Infections, thrombosis, stress ulceration, pressure sores, Addisonian crisis and other medical complications such as pneumonia and ischaemic heart disease. The ultimate prophylactic measure in surgery is to not operate and in every instance it is necessary to consider the risk/benefit ratio even with every possible prophylactic measure.

5. Thromboprophylaxis

What prophylactic measures are available with regard to deep vein thrombosis (DVT)?

Measures which can reduce the risk of thrombosis can be classified as general, physical and chemical.

General measures include: cessation of smoking, avoidance of oestrogen drugs for six weeks pre-operatively, adequate pre-operative hydration, pre-operative weight loss in obese patients, early postoperative mobilisation and avoiding restrictive pressure on calves.

Physical measures include TED (thromboembolic disease) compression stockings and intra-operative pneumatic calf pumping mechanisms.

Chemical measures essentially mean the use of heparin. Low dose, low-molecular-weight heparin is administered subcutaneously in the peri-operative period. This reduces the DVT risk, without significant additional risk of bleeding. Unfractionated heparin is still occasionally used for DVT prophylaxis; it may be easier to reverse with bleeding emergencies. Coumarins (warfarin), indanediones and dextran anticoagulants are not generally used for DVT prophylaxis.

What are the risk factors for DVT?

Previous history of DVT, age, obesity, long operations, pelvic or lower limb surgery, pregnancy, high dose oestrogen therapy, malignancy, heart failure, infections, inflammatory conditions, coagulation disorders including polycythaemia, thrombocythaemia and thrombophilia, and prolonged bed rest.

6. Antibiotic prophylaxis

What prophylactic measures are available with regard to infections?

1.3.6

These can broadly be classified as protecting the patient and protecting the hospital staff. Measures such as aseptic technique (see section 2.5.8) and vaccination against hepatitis B protect both. Procedures specific to preventing infection in patients include isolating elective MRSA-free patients on special wards pre-operatively, skin cleansing, sterile operative procedures, air filtration and channelling, short operations, minimal movement of personnel in and out of theatre and prophylactic antibiotics.

What are the principles of the use of prophylactic antibiotics?

Prophylactic antibiotics are administered to reduce the incidence of postoperative infections. Thus, the antibiotics must be present at effective concentrations throughout the period of risk, they should be bactericidal and they should be appropriate to the sensitivities of the types of organisms likely to be present. They should not be harmful to the patient (allergies should be checked before administration).

Prophylactic antibiotics are used in instances when either the risk of infection is common due to the presence of potentially infective bacteria, e.g. colorectal surgery, or when infection is rare but the consequences are catastrophic, e.g. with implanted orthopaedic or vascular prostheses.

High risk patients can be classified into three groups:

◆ Normal healthy people having contaminated procedures.
◆ Immunocompromised patients.
◆ Patients with anatomical abnormalities such as prosthetic implants or damaged heart valves.

Describe wound classification according to infection risk

Wounds can be classified according to their infection risk into four types.

◆ Clean wounds are those in which there is no contamination from the gut, genitourinary or respiratory tracts, e.g. excision of a skin tumour. The incidence of infection is 1-5%.
◆ Clean-contaminated wounds are those in which there is minimal contamination from the above sources, e.g. removal of the submandibular gland. The incidence of infection is 7-10%.

◆ Contaminated wounds are those in which there is significant risk of contamination, e.g. hemicolectomy. The incidence of infection is 15-20%.

◆ Dirty operations are those which are performed in the presence of infection, e.g. incision and drainage of abscess. The incidence of infection is 30-40%.

7. Pre-medication

What are the objectives of pre-medication drugs?

Pre-medication is the administration of drugs in the hours prior to anaesthesia, to increase the likelihood of the patient of having a smooth, safe anaesthetic. Objectives of pre-medication include anxiety reduction, sedation, amnesia, analgesia, antiemesis, reduction of gastric acid secretion and increase of vagal tone to reduce secretions and reduce gastric motility.

What are the classes of pre-medication drugs?

◆ Benzodiazepines - anxiolytic, sedative and amnesic. May cause over-sedation and respiratory depression. Examples:
  • midazolam, used as pre-medication but also can be administered intravenously for sedation during endoscopy and to reduce distress during procedures performed under local anaesthetic;
  • temazepam, orally 1-2 hours before surgery;
  • diazepam, orally or intravenously.
◆ Opioids - analgesic, anxiolytic and sedative. May cause respiratory depression, e.g. papaveretum (Omnopon™), morphine.
◆ Anticholinergics - used to dry secretions, sedative and antiemetic. May cause bradycardia and confusion, e.g. atropine, glycopyrronium, hyoscine (Scopolamine™).
◆ Antiemetics - e.g. metoclopramide (Maxolon™), prochlorperazine (Stemetil™), ondansetron.
◆ Antacids - to prevent damage from aspiration of gastric contents, e.g. ranitidine, omeprazole.

8. Blood transfusion

How do you estimate a patient's circulating volume?

A healthy adult circulating blood volume is approximately 70ml/Kg. Of this, 40-50% will be cellular and the rest is plasma. If the patient is hypovolaemic they will show signs of hypovolaemic shock (see section 3.11.14).

1.3.8

How do you decide if the patient is likely to need a blood transfusion?

The assessment of what is an adequate pre-operative haemoglobin level for patients undergoing elective surgery should be made on an individual patient basis. It should be based on the clinical condition of the patient and the planned procedure. Accurate estimations of the blood loss and appropriate replacement are necessary to use blood appropriately. However, there are invariably local guidelines available.

Examples of blood requirements for sample operations:

General surgery:

◆ Mastectomy - group and save (G&S).
◆ Cholecystectomy (open/laparoscopic) - (G&S).
◆ Anterior resection (open/laparoscopic) - 2 units.
◆ Oesophagectomy - 4 units.

Vascular surgery:

◆ Abdominal aortic aneurysm (elective) - 4 units.
◆ Abdominal aortic aneurysm (rupture) - 8 units.
◆ Femoral-popliteal bypass - (G&S).
◆ Limb amputation - 2 units.

Orthopaedic surgery:

◆ Total hip/knee replacement - (G&S).
◆ Revision hip/knee surgery - 2 units.
◆ Femoral/tibial nailing - 2 units.

Head and neck:

◆ Thyroidectomy - (G&S).
◆ Tonsillectomy - (G&S).

Urology/gynaecology:

◆ Transurethral resection of prostate - (G&S).
◆ Radical prostatectomy - 4 units.
◆ Nephrectomy - 2 units.
◆ Hysterectomy (abdominal/vaginal) - (G&S).
◆ Caesarean section - (G&S).

Other:

◆ Craniotomy for extradural haemorrhage - 2 units.
◆ Open heart surgery - 6 units.

What is the difference between a 'group and save' (G&S) and a 'cross match'?

A group and save is a request for the laboratory to perform only quick and cheap preliminary tests to 'type' the blood and keep it for further cross matching when, or if, transfusion is required. A cross match is a request for a specified amount of fully tested, cross matched blood for transfusion. It would also specify when the blood is required.

9. Consent

What do you understand by informed consent?

The patient must be competent, consent must be voluntary and there must be sufficient disclosure of information. The information given will depend upon factors such as the nature of the condition and the risks associated with the procedure and the patient's own wishes. For example, patients may need more information about a procedure which carries a high risk of failure or significant complications. The information which should be offered may include: details of the diagnosis, the prognosis, and the likely prognosis if the condition is left untreated, as well as options for management of the condition, which should include the option not to treat. No-one may make decisions on behalf of a competent adult. A patient may ask to have information withheld and for others to make decisions on their behalf, or nominate a relative or third party to make decisions for them.

Consent should be obtained by the person providing treatment or undertaking an investigation, as they will have a comprehensive understanding of the procedure or treatment, how it is carried out, and the risks attached to it. Where this is not practicable, the dentist or doctor may delegate these tasks provided the person to whom the tasks are delegated is suitably trained and qualified and has sufficient knowledge of the proposed investigation or treatment, and understands the risks involved.

Is a signed consent form legal proof that consent was obtained?

No, a signed consent form is not sufficient evidence that a patient has agreed or still agrees to the proposed investigation or treatment, in all its aspects. A member of the healthcare team must review the patient's decision with them at or near to the time of treatment. They must check that the patient still wishes to proceed and respond to any new or further concerns that may arise. This is especially important if there have been changes in the patient's condition.

When do children under the age of 16 have the legal capacity to consent to medical treatment?

Children and young people should be involved as much as possible in discussions about their care, even if they are not able to make decisions on their own. It has been legally established in the Gillick case that children under the age of 16 could give consent independent of their parents' wishes if they had sufficient understanding and intelligence. Therefore, when assessing a young person's capacity to make decisions about investigations or treatment, it should be borne in mind that they may have capacity to make their own decisions, depending on their maturity and ability to understand what is involved. At age 16 a young person can be presumed to have capacity to make most decisions about their care and treatment, although there may be limits on their right to refuse treatment.

10. Pre-operative fasting

Why are patients fasted prior to surgery?

Patients having elective surgery under general anaesthetic require pre-operative fasting, to prevent regurgitation of gastric contents causing aspiration pneumonia. When an endotracheal tube or laryngeal mask is placed, stimulation of the oropharynx can produce gagging, or induce vomiting. In a paralysed patient there is a loss of the normal reflexes preventing aspiration of gastric contents.

What are the usual fasting times?

◆ Adults - six hours nil by mouth to food and milk-containing fluids, four hours nil by mouth to clear fluids, two hours for water.
◆ Reduced fasting time in neonates and children.

1.3.10

Which patients are at high risk of aspiration?

Patients with obesity, pregnancy or ascites, diabetes, gastric reflux, hiatus hernia, depressed consciousness and non-fasted patients, for example, with emergency surgery.

What methods are used to reduce the dangers of aspiration of gastric contents?

Following fasting the patients are usually intubated, or the laryngeal mask placed with the patient slightly head down. Pre-operative administration of antacids or proton pump inhibitors can reduce gastric acidity. In patients with hiatus hernia, or in major abdominal surgery, the airway is protected once a cuffed endotracheal tube is *in situ* with the cuff inflated.

In non-fasted patients, for example, emergency trauma surgery, rapid-sequence induction is performed. The patient is first pre-oxygenated and should always be intubated in the head down position. Cricoid pressure is used to manually depress the cricoid cartilage, effectively occluding the oesophagus to prevent aspiration, whilst endotracheal intubation is performed, after an intravenous induction agent and muscle relaxant have been administered.

11. Preparing the operating list

What information should be on an operating list?

♦ Patient's name.
♦ Hospital ID number.
♦ Date and time of list.
♦ Date of birth/age.
♦ Ward.
♦ Procedure.
♦ Operating surgeon's name.
♦ Anaesthetist's name.

- Theatre number.
- Order on list.
- Relevant comorbidities, e.g. diabetic, latex allergy.
- Infection status, e.g. HIV, MRSA.
- Blood transfusion status, e.g. group and save, cross match two units.
- Other special requirements, e.g. frozen section required, on-table imaging, microscope.

To whom should operating lists be distributed?

- Operating theatre/anaesthetic room.
- Theatre reception.
- Recovery.
- Wards.
- Operating surgeon(s).
- Anaesthetists.
- Theatre scheduler/coding clerks.
- Blood transfusion department.
- Theatre porters.

What factors determine the order of the list?

Most surgeons prefer to perform complex procedures early on the list whilst they are still fresh and not tired, and to allow some 'daylight hours' recovery time. Balanced against this preference are certain other requirements:

- Children - surgery early on list.
- Diabetics - early on list, to reduce long periods of starvation.
- Day surgery hoping to leave hospital same day - early on list to allow plenty of recovery time.
- Dirty cases, e.g. anal surgery - towards end of list.
- Infection risk cases, e.g. HIV, MRSA - towards end of list.

Chapter 4

Pathways and protocols

1. Integrated care pathways (ICP)

What is an ICP?

An ICP is a multi-disciplinary outline of planned care, in an appropriate timeframe, to help a patient with a specific condition or set of symptoms move progressively through a clinical experience to positive outcomes.

Variations from the pathway may occur as clinical freedom is exercised to meet the needs of the individual patient.

When designing and introducing ICPs, it is important to incorporate them into organisational strategy and choose appropriate topics which will provide opportunities for improvement.

What are the advantages of ICPs?

ICPs are important because they help to reduce unnecessary variations in patient care and outcomes. They support the development of care partnerships and empower patients and their carers.

ICPs can also be used as a tool to incorporate local and national guidelines into everyday practice, manage clinical risk and meet the requirements of clinical governance.

Give some examples of ICPs

The success of ICPs can be gauged by looking at the vast number of ICPs in use around the world; there is even a Journal of Integrated Care Pathways. There are pathways for almost every aspect of patient care, from pre-admission clinic to rapid discharge home of the dying patient. There are pathways for management of almost all medical and surgical conditions from rheumatoid arthritis to prostate cancer. There are also many national and international web sites for the development and implementation of ICPs and to help medical professionals develop their own ICPs.

2. Patient identification

What safeguards are used in hospital to safely identify patients?

1.4.2

Each patient should have two identification bands fixed to their wrists or ankles. Where possible they should be asked to confirm their name AND date of birth.

At what times, in particular, is it most important to check patient identification?

When giving drugs: drugs and dosages are checked against the drug chart and if possible by asking the patient. In unconscious patients, the notes, wrist band and drug chart should be checked.

When starting blood transfusion: check the wristband, notes, prescription chart and compatibility label attached to the blood component pack. Check the transfusion compatibility form sent with the blood component pack for name, hospital number, date of birth, ward, hospital, laboratory number, date and time of request, blood group, component unit number, product (e.g. packed red cells, fresh frozen plasma), cross match result (compatibility) and expiry date.

When ordering investigations: check the patient's name and address, hospital ID number, date of birth/age, ward/department, details of request (e.g. ultrasound, blood count), clinical details, consultant, infection status (e.g. HIV, MRSA), signature, date.

At theatre check in: check the patient's wristband for name and address, hospital ID number, date of birth/age. Confirm the ward/department, operation, surgeon, anaesthetist, theatre, infection status (e.g. HIV, MRSA). In addition, the patients are checked for consent, notes, blood results/investigations available, availability of ITU/HDU bed if required, the presence of metal prostheses/pacemakers/dentures/caps/crowns, anti-embolus stockings, jewellery and rings, if on a canvas, hearing aids, make-up and nail varnish removed, nil-by-mouth status, glasses/contact lenses, shaving and pre-operative marking.

3. Clinical governance

Describe what you understand by clinical governance

Clinical governance is corporate responsibility for clinical practice. The definition used in the United Kingdom is: "The framework through which the National Health Service is accountable for the continuing improvement of quality of the service whilst still safeguarding high standards of care, thereby creating an environment which aims for clinical excellence."

Clinical governance incorporates control of the effectiveness of medical care using techniques such as audit and national guidelines, as well as the provision of education and training.

1.4.3

What is audit?

The definition of audit is "The systematic critical analysis of the quality of medical care, including the procedures used for diagnosis and treatment, the use of resources and the resulting outcome and quality of life for the patient".

An audit cycle or circle works by identifying the problem or objective, determining what are the required standards and then collecting data to compare to those standards. When the data are collected for assessment and if the required standard is not attained, then areas of improvement are identified. Changes are made and the audit is repeated to see if changes have raised standards to the required level. The cycle should continue until the required standard is achieved.

How is audit performed in the hospital situation?

Most hospitals have an audit department which advises and assists the audit process. However, many hospital audits begin within clinical departments. The initiating factor is usually a desire to see if patient care can be improved. The first stage of audit design is to determine an aim. The aim is usually based on an aspect of care the team would like to improve. The next step is to see what are the gold standards for that aspect of care. The auditor then needs to find a way of assessing the aspect of care and how it can be compared with the gold standard. This usually requires the audit department's help and a plan is made on how to collect and analyse data. It is important to be certain that the data collected will be relevant to the aim of the audit. This may require a small pilot study first. If the pilot study is successful the data are then collected, analysed and usually presented in an audit meeting. If there is room for improvement in the department's standard of care there is usually a discussion about how the standards can be improved. The changes required are agreed and implemented and the audit cycle is then repeated after a predetermined period of time to see if the changes have been effective.

4. Evidence-based medicine

What do you understand by the term evidence-based medicine (EBM)?

According to the Centre for Evidence-Based Medicine, EBM is the conscientious, explicit and judicious use of current best evidence in making decisions about the care of individual patients. The practice of evidence-based medicine means integrating individual clinical expertise with the best available external clinical evidence from systematic research. Individual clinical expertise means the proficiency and judgement that individual clinicians acquire through clinical experience. Increased expertise is reflected in many ways, but especially in more effective and efficient diagnosis, and in the more thoughtful identification and compassionate use of individual patients' predicaments, rights, and preferences in making clinical decisions about their care. Best available external clinical evidence means clinically relevant research.

External clinical evidence may invalidate previously accepted diagnostic tests and treatments and replaces them with new ones that are more effective and safer.

Name some good sources of up-to-date evidence-based medicine

Quality filtered or summarised evidence-based medicine can be obtained from sources such as the Cochrane Library, the Centre for Evidence-Based Medicine, *The Journal of Evidence-Based Medicine*, *Journal of Evidence-Based Dentistry*, specialist Libraries such as the National Library for Health, Bandolier and any of the large number of specialist centres for evidence-based healthcare, including the Centre for Statistics in Medicine in Oxford, Centre for Evidence-Based Child Health in London, Centre for Evidence-Based Dentistry in Oxford, Centre for Evidence-Based Dermatology in Nottingham and Centre for Evidence-Based Medicine, Mount Sinai, Toronto.

5. Multi-disciplinary meetings (MDM)

What is an MDM?

All patients should be under the care of a multi-disciplinary team. A multi-disciplinary medical team is comprised of healthcare professionals who provide optimal patient care through co-ordination and communication with one another. A multi-disciplinary team provides a continuum of care for patients through diagnosis, treatment, recovery and rehabilitation.

Who are usually present?

Different surgical specialties require different teams. For example, an oncology MDM would involve some or all of the following: surgeons, oncologists, radiologists, histopathologists, cytologists, clinical nurse specialists and allied professions including dentists and physiotherapists, speech and swallowing specialists, nutritionists and palliative care specialists.

Who co-ordinates the MDM?

A dedicated MDM co-ordinator is required to organise and collate input for the meeting.

All discussion should be recorded in the notes and written records disseminated to all members of the team and the general practitioner. Appropriate action can then be arranged.

6. Infection control practices - infections

What are the principles of surgery on a patient known to be a carrier of methicillin-resistant *Staphylococcus aureus* (MRSA)?

If the patient is an outpatient awaiting elective surgery they should have the surgery delayed until they have been demonstrated to be clear of

MRSA. This is not only because known carriers of MRSA are at increased risk of surgical complications themselves but they could also introduce the bacteria to the ward or theatre environment. When the patient is clear of MRSA it may be possible for them to be admitted to a dedicated ward for elective surgery patients who have been swabbed and are proven not to be carriers. This is a common practice for elective orthopaedic surgery, which is clean surgery where the colonisation of prosthetic implants with MRSA can have disastrous results. In emergency situations the benefits of surgery will usually outweigh the risks; however, MRSA may alter the treatment plan. Certainly, placement of implants and skin grafting is generally avoided in known carriers until it is eradicated. MRSA-positive patients are generally placed on the end of operation lists, if possible, and go direct to theatre instead of via a holding bay. Eradication regimens vary from one hospital to another and microbiology advice should be sought if there is any doubt about the best management of these patients.

What blood-borne viruses are of greatest concern to the surgical team?

The hepatitis B and C and, more recently, G viruses and the human immunodeficiency virus (HIV) are of greatest concern to the surgical team as they are transmissible through bodily fluids and may be fatal. Approximately 1-12% of people who are infected with hepatitis B virus (HBV) after birth become chronic carriers. This places them at increased risk of developing liver cancer and a small percent of people die from acute liver failure. About 5-30% of people infected with HCV develop cirrhosis over a long period of time. HGV appears to cause long-term viraemia and as a cofactor seems to make HCV and HBV outcomes worse. It is not yet known if it causes cirrhosis or liver failure.

What vaccinations are available against them?

There are no vaccinations yet against HIV, HCV or HGV. The vaccination against HBV has about 90-95% effectiveness, although persons over 40 years are less likely to respond.

If someone is inoculated with HBV and is not vaccinated they should be given hepatitis B immunoglobulin (HBIG) within 14 days.

7. Infection control practices - universal precautions

What are universal precautions?

The universal precautions were the precautions originally devised when a patient was known to be infected with a blood-borne pathogen. However, since then it has been realised that the surgical team regularly operate on patients who are infected without knowing it and the precautions have become advisory for all cases, i.e. universal. Universal precautions are designed to protect patients and medical staff:

◆ Wash hands before and after every patient contact, and immediately if in direct contact with blood or body fluids, and avoid hand to mouth/ eye contact.

◆ Wear gloves when in contact with blood or body fluids, mucous membranes or non-intact skin is anticipated and wash hands after their removal.

◆ Take precautions to prevent puncture wounds, cuts and abrasions in the presence of blood.

◆ Protect skin lesions and existing wounds by means of waterproof dressings and/or gloves.

◆ Avoid invasive procedures if suffering from chronic skin lesions on the hands.

◆ Avoid use of or exposure to sharps and sharp objects when possible, but when unavoidable, take particular care in their handling and ensure approved procedures are followed for their disposal.

◆ Never re-sheath needles. Always dispose of needles directly into sharps bins.

◆ Protect the eyes and mouth by means of a visor, goggles or safety spectacles and a mask whenever splashing is a possibility.

◆ Wear rubber boots or plastic disposable overshoes when the floor or ground is likely to be contaminated.

◆ Control surface contamination by blood and body fluids through containment and appropriate decontamination procedures.

◆ Use approved procedures for sterilisation and disinfection of instruments and equipment.
◆ Clear up spillages of blood and other body fluids promptly and disinfect surfaces.
◆ Dispose of all contaminated waste and linen safely.
◆ Use the agreed procedure for the safe disposal of contaminated wastes.

8. Infection control practices - needlestick injuries

What is the risk of infection if an operator suffers a needlestick injury which is positive for HIV or HBV?

The risk of acquiring HIV through a contaminated sharps injury is approximately 0.3% for a percutaneous exposure and 0.09% for a mucous membrane exposure. The risk for HBV is much higher at 6-24% for a non-immunised host. For HCV it is 1-10%. Some factors cause a particularly high risk:

◆ Deep puncture or having punctured a blood vessel.
◆ Large bore needles.
◆ 'Donor' patient with terminal HIV (AIDS) infection.
◆ Blood visible on instrument or needle.

What is the protocol following a sharps injury?

Most hospitals have local protocols which should be well displayed and should be familiar to anyone who might come into contact with contaminated sharps.

The general procedures following a contaminated sharps injury are:

◆ Encourage bleeding, wash with soap and running water.
◆ Report the incident and discuss with a local medical expert, such as a Public Health Consultant immediately. They will want to know the type of injury, donor HIV status if known, and your immune status, etc.

If this urgent preliminary risk assessment considers there is a significant risk of HIV, post-exposure prophylaxis (PEP) needs to be started as soon as possible - ideally within one hour. This reduces risk of transmission by 80%. It may be appropriate to give the first dose of PEP pending a fuller assessment after the HIV status of the donor is known. Where the donor is unknown, epidemiological likelihood of HIV in the source needs to be considered, although in most cases PEP will not be justified.

PEP consists of a 28-day course of treatment with a triple combination of antiretroviral drugs. PEP has significant side effects, and needs careful follow-up.

Depending on the health worker's HBV immunisation status consideration should be give to the use of HBV immunoglobulins.

It is usually necessary to arrange for blood samples to be taken from the person who suffered the needlestick injury, as well as the person whose blood was the contaminant on the sharp. Informed consent is important.

Finally, it is usual to fill out the incident book and complete critical event audit. Consideration can then be given to how subsequent events can be prevented.

9. Emergency surgery - principles

What are the principles of the immediate management of any acutely unwell patient?

1.4.9

It is generally acknowledged that the safest method of initial management of any acutely unwell patient, for any cause, is to use a standardised ABCDE approach. This approach is the basis of many courses on the management of acutely unwell patients and has been shown to minimise the chances of overlooking life-threatening conditions and maximises the chance of keeping the patient alive long enough, or stabilising the patient, for expert help to arrive. Details of the ABCDE approach are given in the following questions.

What general methods of trauma management do you know?

Probably the best well known and generally accepted international method for trauma management is the Advanced Trauma Life Support® (ATLS) program which is written by the American College of Surgeons.

Outline the principles of that method

The ATLS program is designed to enable a doctor with basic knowledge to assess a patient's condition reliably and rapidly, to resuscitate and stabilise them, and then determine if the patient needs specialist care and if that care can be provided in house or if the patient needs transfer elsewhere.

The principles of the ATLS program are that the doctor should perform a primary survey using a logical, stepwise approach:

◆ Airway and C-spine immobilisation.
◆ Breathing.
◆ Circulation.
◆ Disability.
◆ Exposure and Environmental control.

At each stage in the primary survey any life-threatening conditions should be identified and managed immediately. When interventions are performed the survey returns each time back to A and the stepwise approach is repeated.

After the primary survey, resuscitation should be well underway and the patient should be showing signs of normalisation. This is followed by a secondary survey which is a head to toe evaluation and includes a complete history, including mechanism of injury and the patient's previous medical history. During the evaluation, extra investigations are obtained and the patient is constantly re-evaluated. After identifying the patient's injuries and providing immediate life-saving care, definitive care begins. This may involve transfer to another department, theatre or another hospital.

10. Emergency surgery - airway

How would you assess a patient's airway?

Maintenance of a patient's airway and adequate oxygen delivery are essential in all patients. All emergency patients should be administered supplemental oxygen.

Signs of acute airway obstruction may be obvious, e.g. coughing, choking, stridor, gurgling, cyanosis, absence of ventilatory effort, or may be more subtle, e.g. tachypnoea, agitation, altered level of consciousness. Other clues include signs of facial or airway trauma, or presence of vomit in or around the mouth.

◆ **Look** - for obstruction in the oral cavity.
◆ **Listen** - for airflow at the mouth and nose; does the airflow give indication of partial obstruction?
◆ **Feel** - for airflow at the mouth and nose.

What is the immediate management of an obstructed airway?

In trauma patients, airway management should always be achieved with immobilisation of the cervical spine to prevent displacement of neck fractures. The mouth is gently opened and any source of obstruction, e.g. tongue, vomit, dentures, broken teeth, secretions, removed directly or with suction. The chin lift and jaw thrust manoeuvres can be performed to maintain airway patency by preventing the tongue and palate from flopping back and causing obstruction. In the unconscious patient an oropharyngeal (Guedel) or nasopharyngeal airway can be inserted to maintain upper airway patency. A supplemental oxygen mask with reservoir bag is then applied.

1.4.10

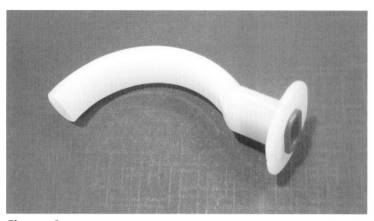

Figure 1. Guedel airway.

What is a definitive airway?

A definitive airway is a safe artificial airway that will maintain patency from the outside, into the trachea beyond the vocal cords. Definitive airways include orotracheal intubation, nasotracheal intubation and a surgical airway, e.g. cricothyroidotomy or tracheostomy (see section 3.10.11). It does not include a laryngeal mask as these do not prevent aspiration and can be easily displaced.

Indications for a definitive airway include:

◆ Inability to maintain airway with the above simple measures.
◆ Apnoea.
◆ Hypoxia despite adequate oxygen delivery by mask.
◆ Protection from impending obstruction, e.g. burns, facial trauma.
◆ Protection from aspiration.
◆ Severe head injury.
◆ Vocal cord paralysis.

11. Emergency surgery - breathing

How do you assess a patient's breathing?

Breathing (ventilation) is the next item to be assessed according to the 'ABC' mantra of emergency resuscitation, after the airway has been secured with cervical spine immobilisation.

Signs of compromised ventilation include cyanosis or tachypnoea in the absence of a compromised airway. The whole thorax needs to be examined for signs of blunt or penetrating injury, and auscultation for adequate air entry is performed over the apices and bases of the lungs. Asymmetrical chest wall movements and tracheal deviation are noted.

◆ **Look** - for cyanosis, laboured breathing and chest and abdominal wall movements, and check the respiratory rate.
◆ **Listen** - for air entry - is it equal?
◆ **Feel** - for chest expansion and percuss for resonance.
◆ **Test** - for oxygen saturation with a pulse oximeter.

What are the causes of reduced ventilation in the trauma patient and how would you manage them?

Haemothorax is due to blood in the chest cavity, usually from rib fractures or lung injury. It may cause reduced chest wall movement with ventilation and may be dull on percussion. Chest X-ray confirms fluid in the chest. Mild/moderate haemothorax is treated with a chest drain (see section 3.10.12), but severe haemothorax with evidence of ongoing bleeding requires urgent surgery.

Simple pneumothorax is due to air in the pleural space, outside the lung, from penetrating trauma or lung damage. It causes reduced chest wall movement with ventilation and may be hyper-resonant on percussion. The trachea may be central or deviated to the side of the pneumothorax. Chest X-ray confirmation is required and significant pneumothoraces are treated with a chest drain.

Tension pneumothorax is an acute surgical emergency, due to air in the pleural space, outside the lung, collecting at high pressure as it can enter the pleural cavity, but not leave due to lung damage acting as a one-way valve. It causes reduced chest wall movement, hyper-resonance and profound tracheal deviation away from the side of the pneumothorax. The high pressure rapidly leads to reduced venous return and cardiac arrest. Chest X-ray confirmation is not required. On suspicion of the diagnosis, treatment is with needle pleurocentesis and then a chest drain is placed later.

12. Emergency surgery - circulation

How would you assess a patient's circulation?

- ◆ **Look** - for altered mental state, sweating, pallor, capillary refill, JVP and respiratory rate.
- ◆ **Listen** - for heart sounds; is there muffling to suggest fluid around the heart?
- ◆ **Feel** - for pulses, proximally and peripherally; what is the rate, character and rhythm?
- ◆ **Test** - for blood pressure, perform an ECG and monitor urine output.

1.4.12

Why is it important to know if the patient is taking beta-blockers?

Patients taking beta-blockers will not show normal tachycardia in response to hypovolaemia and the blood pressure may fall more quickly.

Why might the capillary refill time be prolonged in a patient's finger but not at their sternum?

Capillary refill time is usually two seconds, following compression for five seconds. If the environmental temperature is low the patient may have peripheral capillary bed closure to conserve heat which would affect the finger capillaries more than central capillaries. Other reasons might include compromise to the proximal vascular supply of the finger.

If a patient has lost a quarter of their circulating volume rapidly and a blood sample is taken immediately what will be the change in their haemoglobin concentration?

There will be little or no change in their haemoglobin concentration. It is important to appreciate the limitation of using haemoglobin concentration as an indicator of blood loss, especially in the acute setting. A way to understand this is to imagine instead of looking at haemoglobin concentration in blood measured as grams of haemoglobin per decilitre, we are looking at tadpole concentration in a bucket. The bucket holds 5 litres and there are a 100 tadpoles so the concentration is 100 per 5 litres or 20 per litre. Assuming they are evenly distributed then if you empty half the bucket there will be 50 in 2.5 litres of water which is a concentration of 20 per litre, so there is no change in concentration. The same applies to haemoglobin concentration and blood loss. It is not until the lost blood is replaced by other fluid (which in a trauma situation is a mixture of interstitial fluids and infused colloids and crystalloids) that the concentration falls. In the above example if the bucket is topped-up to five litres with water the concentration will be 50 tadpoles per 5 litres or 10 per litre. It is important to remember that the haemoglobin concentration will not change after blood loss until the circulating volume has been topped up and that takes time.

13. Screening

What are the principles of cancer screening?

The disease being screened for should have a high prevalence and incidence in the screened population. Screening should have benefits in terms of reduced mortality and morbidity, and reduced social and financial costs. The biology and natural history of the disease should be

1.4.13

understood; the cancer should exist for a long time in a preclinical phase when screening can detect it and this preclinical phase should have a high prevalence rate in the screened population to make the testing worthwhile. The disease should have an effective treatment at an early stage, and this treatment should be more effective than treatment at a late stage, otherwise it defeats the object of screening.

An effective screening test should have the ability to detect cancer in its preclinical phase with high levels of accuracy (sensitivity, specificity and predictive values). The test should be safe and socially acceptable. If the screened individuals are asymptomatic they will not co-operate if they could suffer complications of a screening examination. To be applied efficiently in large populations, the screening test should be simple, inexpensive and accessible.

The most important outcome measure of the effectiveness of a screening strategy is the demonstration that the mortality rate from the disease is significantly lower in the total screened population when compared with the mortality rate in an equivalent population of unscreened people, preferably demonstrated by a randomised, controlled, defined population clinical trial.

What screening programs do you know?

There are several cancer screening programs, including breast cancer screening by mammography for women between 50 and 70 years, cervical cancer screening is offered to women between 25 and 64 years, and a colorectal cancer screening program is being offered to men and women between 60 and 69 years in some areas. Screening for abdominal aortic aneurysm has been shown to be effective, but is not yet widely implemented.

14. Surgical oncology

1.4.14

What are carcinogens, initiators and promoters?

A carcinogen is a cancer-causing substance or agent. They can be classified as chemical, viral, radiation, hormones, mycotoxins, parasites and miscellaneous agents, such as asbestos.

Examples of chemical carcinogens are aromatic amines which cause bladder cancer, alkylating agents which cause leukemia and azo-dyes which cause bladder and liver cancer. Viral carcinogens include human papilloma virus (HPV), implicated in cervical and oral carcinoma, Epstein Barr virus (EBV) in nasopharyngeal carcinoma, and hepatitis B virus (HBV) which causes hepatocellular carcinoma. Non-ionizing radiation is implicated in melanoma and non-melanoma skin cancer. Ionizing radiation is implicated in thyroid carcinoma. Hormonal carcinogens include anabolic steroids which are known to cause liver cancer. Oestrogen is implicated in breast cancer. Of the mycotoxins, the best known are the aflatoxins produced by *Aspergillus flavus* which causes liver cancer. Parasitic carcinogens include Schistosoma which causes bladder cancer. Asbestos is in the miscellaneous group and is well known as the major cause of pleural mesothelioma; it also increases the risk of other lung carcinomas especially in cigarette smokers.

The initiator-promoter concept is part of the multi-step theory of carcinogenesis. Initiation is the event that changes the cell's DNA and promotion is the event that stimulates proliferation of the abnormal cell. A promoter affects normal and initiated cells, and causes altered gene expression leading to increased cell proliferation. Initiated and promoted cells can become cancerous, although initiation can do it alone and some initiated cells may need several promoters. For example, in oral squamous cell carcinoma (OSCC) it is thought that tobacco smoke is the initiator and alcohol acts as a promoter. For this reason OSCC is much more common in persons who drink alcohol and smoke but can also occur in those who only smoke or drink. It rarely occurs in those who do neither and in these cases there is probably an unusual cause, such as a genetic predisposition in combination with other carcinogens such as HPV.

What is cancer staging?

A system to formalise datasets so there can be no ambiguity in histological reporting, evaluating treatments and interpreting clinical trials. It also guides management and gives an indication of prognosis.

The TNM staging system was developed in the 1950s:

◆ T is the size and local extent of the primary tumour. TX means it cannot be assessed, T0 means there is no evidence of a primary tumour, e.g. occult primary, Tis means tumour *in situ* and T1-T4 are varying sizes of tumour depending on which type of tumour the system is used for.

◆ N is the presence of regional lymph node metastases. NX means the nodes cannot be assessed, N0 no nodes and N1- N3 varying degrees of nodes depending on the type of tumour.

◆ M is the presence of distant metastases. MX means it cannot be assessed, M0 implies no metastases and M1 distant metastases.

15. Epidemiology

What is the role of epidemiological studies and cancer registration?

Epidemiology has been a useful way of discovering the causes of cancers. It is usual for epidemiologists to analyse cancer incidence rather than mortality, as mortality registers are generally unreliable and not all cancers are fatal. In developed countries the cancer registries are a good source of the required data. In underdeveloped countries it is usually necessary to visit the country and study the population. By analysing variations in tumour incidence within and between populations it can provide clues as to the causes of cancer.

Cancer registries are unique in being able to provide adequate historical trend and population-based data to monitor changes in cancer incidence or survival over long periods of time. Historically, the role of the cancer registries has been to collect population-based data on the incidence of, and survival from, all cancers.

Cancer registries have a critical role in the implementation and monitoring of key national initiatives, such as the NHS cancer plan in England, which aim to improve the quality of care and survival prospects for cancer patients.

Cancer registries also undertake a range of public health surveillance and health protection functions, with cancer registration information being specifically used to:

◆ Monitor trends in cancer incidence, prevalence and survival with time and among different areas and social groups. Differences in cancer incidence, survival and access to treatment among social groups can contribute to programs aimed at reducing inequalities in health outcomes.

◆ Evaluate the effectiveness of cancer prevention and screening programs; for example, to monitor the effectiveness of the existing screening programs in the UK for breast and cervical cancer, and to inform the design of new programs such as screening for colorectal and ovarian cancer.

◆ Evaluate the quality and outcomes of cancer care, through the provision of comparative data on treatment patterns and outcomes.

◆ Evaluate the effect of environmental and social factors on cancer risk and support other investigations into the causes of cancer. Cancer registration information is currently being used, for example, to investigate cancer risks in relation to power lines, landfill sites and mobile phones.

◆ Support the work of cancer genetic counselling services for individuals and families who have a higher risk of developing cancer.

◆ Support recalls of specific groups of cancer patients, for example, women who were treated for Hodgkin's disease with radiotherapy and may have an increased risk of developing breast cancer.

Give some examples where it has changed cancer outcomes

Probably the most famous and earliest example of epidemiology in action is the story of Percival Pott observing in 1777 that scrotal carcinoma is more common in chimney sweeps. He postulated that the soot was responsible. The polycyclic hydrocarbon was isolated 150 years later.

Another more recent example of epidemiology at work in cancer care is the finding that although hepatocellular carcinoma is rare in the developed world it is common in underdeveloped countries. Epidemiology showed that it was common in areas where the incidence of HBV and HCV are high and where there are high levels of mycotoxins. This led to the discovery that food contaminated with aflatoxins from *Apsergillus flavus* is highly carcinogenic. This situation was further compounded by the discovery that HBV is also carcinogenic and it may be that that the aflatoxin causes a mutation in p53, a tumour suppressor gene.

Section 2

The operating theatre environment

Chapter 5

Theatre design and function

1. Operating theatres

Describe the rooms which form a theatre suite, their relations and functions

◆ Operating theatre - this is the hub of the theatre suite and needs to be surrounded by various other areas to facilitate access: anaesthetic room, scrub room, prep room, sluice and instrument/suture store. It is where the actual operations are performed, and needs to be large enough for the operating table, three/four surgeons, scrub nurses, runners, instrument trolleys, anaesthetist(s), anaesthetic assistant, operating department assistant, monitoring equipment, imaging equipment, resuscitation equipment, computer station and students.

◆ Anaesthetic room - where the anaesthetic is administered. It should lie between the holding bay/clean corridor and the operating theatre.

◆ Scrub room - where the surgeons and scrub nurses 'scrub up', clean and disinfect hands, and don gloves and gowns. It should be adjacent to the operating theatre. Scrubbed staff should be able to pass from the scrub room to the theatre without manually opening doors. There is usually no door between the scrub room and the theatre, but sometimes there may be an automatic door, or a foot-operated door.

◆   Preparation room - where the instrument trolleys are prepared and laid out by the scrub nurses. It should be adjacent to the operating theatre.

◆   Recovery - where the patients are monitored postoperatively prior to transfer back to the ward. It is usually adjacent to the clean corridor, and away from the holding bay.

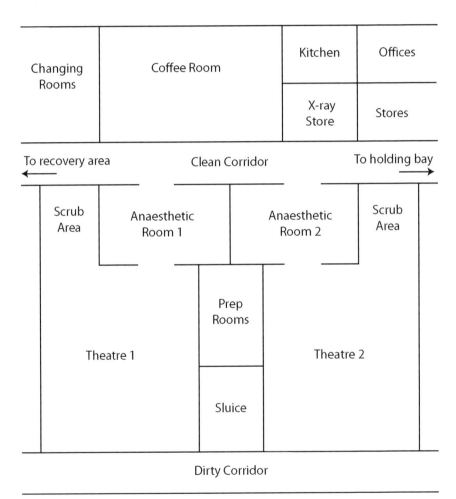

Figure 1. Operating theatre design.

◆ Sluice - a room where used instruments and trays are washed before sending for re-sterilisation, and where 'dirty' liquids are disposed of. It should lie between the operating theatre and the dirty corridor.

◆ Holding bay - where patients are received to the theatre suite, checked in and wait prior to transfer to the anaesthetic room. It should be adjacent to the clean corridor and away from recovery.

◆ Clean corridor - the corridor connecting the anaesthetic room, theatres, changing rooms, recovery and holding bay.

◆ Dirty corridor - the corridor connecting the operating theatres, sluice and central sterile supplies unit or stores.

◆ Other areas - changing rooms, store rooms, offices, recreation/coffee room, kitchen.

Where in a hospital are the operating theatres best situated?

Close to the surgical wards, high dependency unit (HDU), intensive care unit (ITU), accident and emergency department (A&E), Radiology/CT and Sterile Supplies Unit. Ideally, theatres, A&E, ITU and CT should be on the same floor, as elevators are not safe places for unstable surgical patients.

What staff are essential for the safe running of an operating theatre?

Surgeon(s), surgical assistant(s), scrub nurses, runners, anaesthetist(s), anaesthetic assistant, operating department practitioner (ODP) or assistant (ODA) (also called theatre support workers) and a portering and messaging service.

An ODP is a person trained to work in theatre in the scrub, anaesthetic assistant or recovery roles.

2. Scrubbing up

2.5.2

Explain the key features of 'scrubbing up'

Prior to scrubbing, the hands should be 'socially clean', with short clean fingernails. Theatre blues/greens tops and bottoms, or dress, should be worn with bleeps or phones removed from the pockets or turned off. Hair should be tied up and placed in a theatre hat, and clean theatre shoes or clogs worn on the feet. Beards should be clean and trimmed, and a theatre hat with sides for covering beards worn.

When scrubbing up, first, the nails are cleaned with a nail cleaner and under the nails scrubbed with a clean brush. The hands are lathered to above the elbow with a suitable antiseptic scrub solution, e.g. povidone-iodine (Betadine™) or chlorhexidine (Hibiscrub™) wash. The hands and forearms are scrubbed with a soft bristle brush, paying special attention to areas commonly missed: the nails, finger-pads, between the fingers and around the wrists. Recommended scrub time is two minutes. The hands and arms are then rinsed, distally to proximally, under running water and the process repeated.

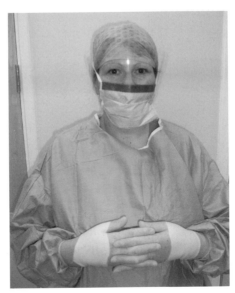

Figure 2. Theatre scrubs.

The gown is lifted from its sterile pack, and donned, without touching the outside of the gown. The ties are secured at the back by an assistant, before the gloves are put on using the 'no-touch technique', so the outside of the gloves are not touched by the scrubbed hands. Finally, the waist tie is secured to cover the buttocks and back.

3. Gloves

Why do surgeons wear gloves?

Surgical gloves are used to protect the patient from infection transmitted from the surgeon, or scrub nurse's hands. Gloves also protect the surgeon from exposure to the patient's body fluids. Some surgeons use double gloving for extra protection.

What types of surgical glove do you know?

- Non-sterile gloves - used for potentially dirty examinations, e.g. rectal or oral examinations. Available in large/medium/small.
- Conventional sterile latex gloves - used for most operations. Available size 5 (very small) to 12 (gorilla!). Can be textured or smooth, powdered or powder-free.
- Non-latex sterile gloves - used when the patient or surgeon suffers from a latex allergy.
- Textured sterile gloves - slightly more grip, e.g. for cardiovascular surgery.
- Powdered gloves - have a fine layer of talc inside to facilitate donning. There is some evidence, however, that talc may cause intra-abdominal adhesions, so some surgeons prefer powder-free gloves. Powdered gloves are also no longer widely used as they may exacerbate the risks of latex allergy.
- Super-sensitive gloves - extra thin. Increased sensitivity for plastic, ophthalmic or paediatric surgery, but not as strong.
- Indicator gloves - have a special mechanism to indicate glove perforation, which works by changing colour when the inside contacts body fluid, or by completing an electric circuit so a buzzer rings. Used for ultra-clean orthopaedic surgery.

2.5.3

4. Masks, goggles and magnification

Why do scrub staff wear masks?

Various trials have shown no benefit for wearing masks in theatre. However, many surgeons continue to wear them, particularly for ultra-clean surgery where surgical prostheses are to be implanted, e.g. vascular surgery, orthopaedic surgery. Surgical masks may even increase infection rates, by rubbing off skin flakes.

However, there is no doubt that masks are beneficial by deflecting forceful expulsion of bacteria-carrying secretions, e.g. cough/sneeze and preventing bogies from falling from the surgeon's nose into the wound!

What should one do in the event of a sneeze whilst wearing a mask in theatre?

Normal practice is to step back from the operating table, but not to face away as this stops secretions being deflected back around the sides of the mask towards the wound.

Why do scrub staff wear goggles?

Goggles are worn simply to prevent contamination of eyes or surrounding mucous membranes from body fluids and debris (e.g. bone fragments in orthopaedic surgery, tooth fragments in dental drilling), which can be splashed or sprayed during surgery. Good quality goggles do not impede the surgeon's vision. Some goggles can be in the form of a visor attached to the surgical mask or combined with magnification devices.

What sources of magnification are available to the surgeon?

Surgical loupes or a microscope. Loupes are cheaper than a microscope but cannot achieve as high a magnification. Loupes are generally easier to use and allow more surgical mobility. The microscope is cumbersome, may be more difficult to use and expensive, but it has an integral light source and can achieve very high magnification. It also allows the assistant to see the operative field through the same lens.

5. Skin preparation and surgical drapes

How and why is skin prepared prior to surgical incision?

Skin preparation solutions are used to 'paint' the skin prior to incision to reduce the risk of infection from skin commensal bacteria and other bacteria, fungi or spores.

Various skin preparations are available. Commonly used are Betadine™, an iodine-based solution, which can be aqueous or alcoholic, chlorhexidine and spirit (an alcohol solution).

Alcohol-based preparations have better bacteriocidal properties but may wash off pre-operative skin marking, and are flammable with a risk of ignition following diathermy spark. Some patients may be allergic to iodine preparations.

Why is the skin shaved prior to surgical incision?

Pre-operative shaving is performed to physically remove hair from the operative field, to remove bacteria carried on hair and to prevent hair tangling with sutures or lying in the wound at skin closure.

There is some evidence that pre-operative shaving can cause skin abrasion increasing infection rates, so depilation is best performed immediately prior to incision, or can be performed using depilatory creams.

What are the principles behind the use of surgical drapes?

Surgical drapes are designed to be a sterile covering around the operative field to prevent contamination of the surgical site from the patient, their clothing and the operating table. They also help to prevent blood and other bodily fluids from contaminating the patient and the clothing. They also may aid in maintaining the patient's body temperature.

Adhesive wound drapes are large clear plastic sheets applied to the skin prior to surgery. The skin is incised through the plastic cover. They may reduce wound contamination and are convenient for keeping hair out of wounds and protecting the skin.

6. Instrument sterilisation

How are surgical instruments sterilised?

Following a surgical procedure, all the instruments are physically cleaned, counted and the sharps (blades/needles) removed. They are then re-packed on to sets for sterilisation. A note is made of any missing, damaged or blunt instruments.

Sterilisation is the complete destruction of all micro-organisms, including bacteria, spores, fungi and viruses. Surgical instrument packs are usually sterilised in an autoclave, which works by high pressure, saturated steam sterilisation. Various sterilisation programs exist, e.g. 130°C, 2.6 bar (37psi) for 20 minutes. The steam penetrates porous wraps to sterilise the contents of the pack. Sterilised packs can be distinguished from non-autoclaved packs by an indicator tape around the pack (Bowie-Dick tape). The lines on the tape become visible following sterilisation. Smaller portable autoclaves are also available for individually wrapped instruments.

What alternative methods of sterilisation do you know?

◆ Dry heat sterilisation - involves heating instruments to 160° for two hours in a hot air oven. It is useful for moisture-sensitive instrument sterilisation, or for instruments with fine cutting edges. Sterilisation is monitored by Brown's tubes, which change colour following exposure to adequate heat.

◆ Ethylene oxide sterilisation - works by exposing items to ethylene oxide gas. It is useful for heat-sensitive equipment (rubber/plastics, etc.), as it is performed at normal temperatures and pressures. It is predominantly used for industrial sterilisation, e.g. sutures, pre-packed catheters, etc.

◆ Gamma ray irradiation - industrial process used for sterilising single-use items, e.g. syringes, catheters.

7. Sterilisation and disinfection

What is the difference between sterilisation and disinfection?

Sterilisation is the complete eradication of all viable micro-organisms including spores and viruses. Disinfection is the reduction in number of organisms; some viruses and spores may remain viable. Although disinfection is not as effective as sterilisation, it is more practical as it does not damage tissues, and can be used for cleaning skin, wiping down surfaces, cleaning floors, etc.

Give some examples of commonly used disinfectants and their applications

◆ Alcohol preparations - effective against all bacteria, some viruses, but not spores or fungi. Work by osmotic effect, denaturing bacteria or viral proteins. Mainly used for skin preparation, but may cause hypersensitivity, or explosions with diathermy (see section 2.7.8).

◆ Chlorhexidine - effective against most bacteria, but not viruses, spores or fungi. Works by bacterial cell wall disruption. Used mixed with detergent for scrubbing up (Hibiscrub™), for wound cleaning (Savlon™), for skin preparation and as a mouthwash.

◆ Iodine-based solutions - good activity against bacteria, spores and fungi, but easily inactivated by body fluids. May cause skin/clothing staining and hypersensitivity reactions. Used for skin preparation, scrubbing up and wound cleansing (Betadine™).

◆ Aldehydes (glutaraldehyde/formaldehyde) - good activity against bacteria and viruses, but needs prolonged exposure for spore and fungi destruction. Causes nasty sensitivity in eyes, skin, mucous membranes. Used for sterilising endoscopes.

8. Aseptic technique

What is aseptic technique?

2.5.8

This is the term for the series of manoeuvres performed to reduce the chances of a surgical wound becoming contaminated. It involves minimising the contact between dirty, clean and sterile objects in the operating theatre environment. It is best described in the following stages:

◆ Scrubbing up - to clean and decontaminate hands and arms (see section 2.5.2).

◆ Donning gown and gloves - is done so the outside of the gown and gloves does not come into contact with the skin or clothes of the person within (see section 2.5.2). When wearing a sterile gown and gloves, the hands are kept at the front, and above the waist.

◆ Patient preparation - the skin is prepped from the centre of the exposed area outward, to reduce the spread of bacteria. Dirty areas (groin, genitalia, anus) are prepped last.

◆ Drape application - drapes are applied to the patient so the sterile operating field does not contact parts of the drapes that have contacted un-prepped parts of the patient.

◆ Trolleys and instruments - care is required to ensure sterile trays and instruments do not contact non-sterile objects; for example, the back of the gown needs to be done up to prevent touching instrument trays which may be behind the surgeon or scrub staff.

- No touch technique - in some ultra-clean procedures, e.g. orthopaedics and vascular, surgeons will try to touch only the tissues with instruments and sutures that have not directly touched the scrub staff or the surgeons' gloves.
- Theatre clean air circulation system - operating theatres are ventilated with filtered and cooled (or warmed) air at a slightly higher pressure than the surrounding rooms. The air enters through vents at the ceiling level, and escapes through slats at floor level in the wall or door of the theatre. Some orthopaedic theatres have ultra-clean air systems, called 'laminar flow', where surgery is performed in a tent ventilated by 'ultra-filtered' air, and the surgeon wears a special clean-suit with an air-exhaust system.

9. The anaesthetic machine

What is an anaesthetic machine?

A portable anaesthesia delivery system that has three functions:

- Delivers anaesthetic gases and oxygen.
- Provides monitoring functions.
- Ventilates patient.

General anaesthesia requires the supply of gases; volatile anaesthetic agents and oxygen. A gas mixture is usually part of the maintenance phase of anaesthesia. Early anaesthetic machines were the original apparatus to deliver anaesthetic gas mixture in a safe and controlled manner. The most famous name in anaesthetic machines is Edmund Boyle who was the first to describe a portable machine for the delivery of oxygen and nitrous oxide in 1917. Modified Boyle's machines are still in use today.

Modern anaesthetic machines have additional functions; as well as being a portable system to deliver anaesthetic volatile agents and oxygen, they mechanically ventilate the patient and provide monitoring functions. The anaesthetic machine usually takes the form of an upright trolley, with monitors at the top, volatile anaesthetic vaporisers in the middle, and the ventilator system at the bottom or on the side. It needs connection to an electricity supply, piped gases, suction and the scavenger system.

2.5.9

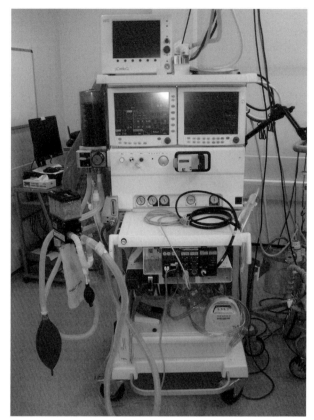

Figure 3. Anaesthetic machine.

What is a scavenger?

A scavenger transfers exhaust gases from the breathing circuit to the hospital exhaust system. This reduces exposure of operating room personnel to anaesthetic pollution which may cause headaches, fatigue, listlessness and may be teratogenic. Scavenger systems may be active or passive.

Passive systems rely on the patients' expiration to force expired anaesthetic gases through a series of pipes into the outside environment. The hazards of this are obstruction or backflow.

Active systems use low pressure suction to remove the gases. These are more complex and there is a potential danger to the patient caused by very low pressures in the anaesthetic circuit. Suction pumps can also be damaged by the volatile anaesthetic agents.

10. Operating table

Describe the essential features of an operating table

◆ Strong and stable - must be able to support the full weight of the patient at any point on the table surface. The maximum supportable weight needs to be clearly written on the table. A heavy base adds to stability to prevent tipping.

◆ Adjustable - must be able to adjust the table to suit all sizes and shapes of patients, operating positions and preferences of the operating team. Electrical systems have the advantage that they can be adjusted without having to reach under drapes but hand-operated systems are cheaper and less likely to malfunction.

◆ Adaptable - need to be able to add on arm boards, head rests and even split the table.

◆ Hygienic - must be easy to clean with disinfectants without dissolving the rubber. Removable parts help with cleaning and must be designed with minimal dirt traps.

◆ Manoeuvrable - often it is necessary to move the operating table. They usually have castor wheels which are lockable.

◆ Pressure area care - rubber cushions should be well padded and replaceable when they are worn.

◆ Radiolucent - it may be necessary to take on-table radiographs or use the image intensifier. If the table is not radiolucent this should be clearly marked on the table.

◆ Insulated - the table should be electrically insulated.

◆ Cost effective - the table should be reparable, and broken or worn parts should be easily replaceable.

2.5.10

11. Patient positioning

Describe the common patient positions for surgery

2.5.11

◆ Supine (on back/face up) - used for most abdominal, groin and chest surgery where exposure from the anterior side is required, e.g. laparotomy, hernia repair, median sternotomy.

◆ Head up - used for many head and neck operations as it reduces filling of the superficial veins, e.g. head up 30° with neck extended for thyroid surgery.

◆ Head down - empties the superficial veins for lower limb surgery, e.g. 30° head down with legs on a vein board for varicose vein surgery.

◆ Prone (on front/face down) - used for posterior approaches, e.g. laminectomy, short saphenous varicose vein surgery.

◆ Lithotomy - supine with the legs up to allow access to the perineum and the abdomen, e.g. anterior resection, haemorrhoidectomy.

◆ Lateral - to allow for approaches from the side, e.g. nephrectomy, thoracotomy.

◆ Sitting - used for some neurosurgical procedures.

What are the complications of different positions?

The patient should always be positioned to minimise risk of intra-operative injury (see section 2.6.9). Different positions may be associated with different complications:

◆ Prone - needs armoured tube to protect airway and special pressure area care.

◆ Lithotomy - may cause hip dislocation, and peroneal nerve palsy.

◆ Head up - air embolus. This occurs as the normal venous pressure in the great veins can be below atmospheric pressure, so in the head up position air can be sucked into the veins.

◆ Head down - may cause diaphragmatic 'splinting', increasing ventilatory pressures in obese patients.

Chapter 6

Anaesthesia

1. Types of anaesthetic

What is an anaesthetic?

An anaesthetic is a drug which renders part (local anaesthetic) or all (general anaesthetic) of the body insensate to pain to allow surgical procedures.

What types of anaesthetic are there and what are the advantages and disadvantages of each?

◆ General anaesthetic. The controlled and reversible induction and maintenance of unconsciousness and analgesia with or without muscle relaxation:
  ● advantages - generally safe and simple. The patient has no pain and no recollection of the experience, and the surgeon has ideal operating conditions;
  ● disadvantages - sometimes unsafe for patients with severe systemic cardiovascular or respiratory disease. There may be an occasional reaction to anaesthetic drugs (allergy, malignant hyperpyrexia).

- Local anaesthetic (see section 2.6.6). Direct administration to operative site (field block):
  - advantages - avoids general anaesthetic. Simple, safe and effective. It is cheap and requires minimal intra-operative monitoring;
  - disadvantages - not suitable for major abdominal/thoracic surgery. Sometimes the block is unsatisfactory and the patient may experience pain. An overdose or inadvertent intravenous administration may cause toxicity.
- Regional block. This form of local anaesthetic is performed by infiltration around sensory nerves remote from the operative site, e.g. ring block by infiltration of digital nerves, for in-growing toenail surgery; inferior alveolar nerve block for dental surgery:
  - advantages - avoids general anaesthetic. It is an effective analgesia if correctly infiltrated, requiring lower volumes of anaesthetic;
  - disadvantages - may be technically difficult to administer. There is a higher risk of inadequate analgesia, inadvertent intravenous administration and direct nerve damage.
- Spinal and epidural anaesthesia (see section 2.6.5):
  - advantages - rapidly effective operative and postoperative analgesia. Avoids general anaesthesia;
  - disadvantages - may be difficult to administer, especially in patients with arthritic spines. It is not suitable in anticoagulated patients and may cause toxicity, hypotension, backache, infection and urinary retention. High blocks may cause respiratory muscle paralysis.

2. General anaesthesia

What are the stages in the administration of a general anaesthetic?

- Pre-operative preparation - (see Chapter 3).
- Induction. The administration of drugs to render the patient unconscious, prior to anaesthetic maintenance and commencing surgery. Intravenous induction agents are quicker and more reliable, but require intravenous access so sometimes induction may be performed using inhalational (maintenance) anaesthetics, e.g. in children. Intravenous induction agents include propofol and etomidate.

- Muscle relaxants. Used for paralysing the patient for anaesthesia where muscle relaxation is required, e.g. major abdominal surgery, or to allow intubation. The patient will require ventilation. There are two types:
  - depolarising muscle agents, e.g. suxamethonium, have a rapid onset and short duration, and work by maintaining the muscle in a relaxed, depolarised state;
  - non-depolarising muscle relaxants, e.g. atracurium, have a slower onset and longer duration, and work by direct non-depolarising neuromuscular blockade.
- Maintenance anaesthetics. Usually inhalational agents, for keeping a patient anaesthetised after induction with intravenous agents. These are administered as a gas mixed with oxygen, via a face mask, laryngeal mask or endotracheal tube, e.g. isoflurane, sevoflurane and desflurane. Halothane is no longer widely used due to risk of liver damage. Maintenance of anaesthesia can also be obtained by direct slow, target-controlled infusion of the intravenous induction agents.
- Recovery (see section 3.9.1).
- Postoperative monitoring (see section 3.9.1).

3. Anaesthetic monitoring

What physiological monitoring is required for a patient undergoing general anaesthetic?

- Pulse rate - can be obtained from ECG monitoring equipment, pulse oximetry or invasive intra-arterial blood pressure monitoring (arterial line).
- ECG monitoring - continuous monitoring from chest leads to display panel. Standard lead II is the best indicator for detecting arrhythmias and ischaemia.
- Blood pressure - may be measured indirectly by manual or automatic dynamap sphygmomanometry or directly by intra-arterial pressure monitoring via a catheter placed in a peripheral artery, usually the radial artery. Continuous direct arterial blood pressure monitoring is required for major cardiothoracic, neurosurgery, vascular surgery or in critically ill or shocked patients.

2.6.3

◆ Pulse oximetry - (see section 2.6.4).

◆ Ventilation monitoring - inspired gas mixture oxygen content monitoring, with oxygen supply failure alarm, tidal/minute volume measurement, ventilator disconnection alarm, and end tidal CO_2 monitoring via capnography with a moving trace.

◆ Urine output - a good indication of renal perfusion and hence overall fluid balance. Essential for major cardiac/vascular/general surgery, in shocked patients or in cases with excess blood or fluid loss.

◆ Central venous pressure measurement - via a subclavian or internal jugular vein (see secion 2.7.2). Provides estimation of circulating fluid volume. Used in major surgery, critically ill patients or patients with cardiac comorbidity. Wedge pressure (pulmonary artery occlusion pressure) measurement is also occasionally useful for patients with cardiac comorbidity as an estimate of filling.

◆ Cardiac output monitoring - this is increasingly used for complex cases or critically ill patients. It can be estimated by pulse contour analysis (PICCO), oesophageal Doppler or by a pulmonary artery catheter (see above).

◆ Temperature measurement - especially for long operations, to prevent hypothermia.

4. Pulse oximetry

What is a pulse oximeter and how does it work?

A pulse oximeter is an electric probe and monitor used to measure arterial oxygen saturation (SaO_2). It does not measure the partial pressure of oxygen (PaO_2) in the blood.

It works by emitting pulses of infrared and visible red light through the tissues and measuring how much is absorbed. Absorption is fairly constant through skin, fat and venous blood, but changing amounts of light are absorbed by pulsatile arterial blood. As oxygenated and deoxygenated blood absorb different amounts of light, the machine is able to calculate a ratio of oxygenated to de-oxygenated blood, and hence estimate SaO_2. The probe takes the form of a clip, with infrared and visible red emitters

2.6.4

on one side and detectors on the other which is clipped across a thin strip of tissue, e.g. finger or ear lobe.

What are the limitations of pulse oximetry?

Pulse oximetry only estimates oxygenation and not ventilation (which is better assessed using pCO_2 estimation). There may be significant delays between SaO_2 and PaO_2 fluctuations. This is due to pulse oximetry calculations being based on a number of pulses rather than being instantaneous and to some extent due to the haemoglobin dissociation curve which may show a significant fall in PaO_2 before SaO_2 decreases.

Pulse oximetry SaO_2 estimation may also be affected by:

- Poor tissue perfusion - shock, hypotension, vasoconstriction - causes no trace.
- Abnormal pulses, e.g. atrial fibrillation
- Movement, e.g. shivering.
- Electrical interference, e.g. diathermy.
- Poor light diffusion, e.g. with nail varnish.
- Abnormal haemoglobin or pigments, e.g. carbon monoxide poisoning - causes a high reading.

It is not normally affected by skin pigmentation.

5. Spinal and epidural anaesthesia

What is the difference between spinal and epidural anaesthesia?

'Spinals' and 'epidurals' are types of regional anaesthesia used to render the lower parts of the body insensate for surgical procedures. Spinal anaesthesia is performed by introducing a needle into the subarachnoid or spinal space and administering drugs, usually a single bolus. Epidural anaesthesia is performed by introducing a catheter into the epidural or extradural space, for administration of drugs as a single bolus

2.6.5

or continuous infusion. Spinal anaesthesia requires a much lower dose than epidural anaesthesia.

These approaches can be used for the administration of local anaesthetics or opiates.

What are the advantages of spinals or epidurals?

These techniques are often safer than general anaesthesia in patients with cardiac or respiratory problems. However, spinal and epidural anaesthesia is contraindicated in patients with aortic stenosis, as the peripheral vasodilation caused can precipitate catastrophic loss of coronary perfusion leading to cardiac ischaemia. This can be mitigated to some extent by intravenous fluid loading and cautious use of vasopressors. A spinal anaesthetic is low dose, low volume, rapid-onset and lasts 1-3 hours. Epidural catheters can be used to infuse higher doses and volumes, and can be used for continuous infusions providing pain relief for 3-4 days.

What are the complications?

Anaesthetic toxicity/overdose, hypotension, headaches, urinary retention, backache, infection, haematoma, abscess, and nerve damage. Epidural anaesthesia can also cause dural tap, a persistent leak of cerebrospinal fluid, which causes severe headache, and may lead to infection. Total spinal is where a large volume of local anaesthetic for an epidural is inadvertently delivered into the subarachnoid space.

6. Local anaesthesia

What local anaesthetics (LA) do you know?

◆   Lidocaine (lignocaine) - the best known LA. Widely used by local subcutaneous infiltration, for nerve blocks, or topically as EMLA™ cream.

2.6.6

◆ Bupivacaine (Marcain™) - slower onset than lidocaine, but longer duration of action, due to tissue binding. Used principally for spinals and epidurals.

◆ Chirocaine - a stereoisomer of bupivacaine that has a lower toxicity.

◆ Prilocaine - lower toxicity than lidocaine. Used for Bier's block (see section 2.6.7).

◆ Cocaine - readily penetrates mucous membranes and has a vasoconstrictor effect. Used for intranasal anaesthesia, too toxic for systemic administration.

How do local anaesthetics work?

Local anaesthetics are solutions, which are infiltrated into tissues or around nerves to render parts of the body insensate to pain for surgical procedures. They work by blockade of sodium channels in cell membranes altering the membrane permeability to block nerve impulses. They are ideal for patients or operations unsuitable for general anaesthesia, as when administered correctly they have a low toxicity, rapid onset and long duration.

Why are they often mixed with vasoconstrictors?

They are often mixed with adrenaline (epinephrine) (usually 1:200,000 [marcaine] or 1:80,000 [lignocaine]) as this causes local vasoconstriction, preventing the systemic distribution of the agents and thus prolonging duration. Local anaesthesia with adrenaline (epinephrine) should not be used in extremities, e.g. fingers, genitalia, due to the risk of profound vasoconstriction leading to ischaemic extremities. Care should be taken in patients with ischaemic heart disease and arrhythmias.

What are the symptoms and signs of systemic toxicity?

Toxicity can occur from inadvertent intravenous administration or overdosage. Early symptoms include peri-oral tingling, paraesthesia, anxiety and drowsiness. This may later progress to cardiac arrhythmias, seizures, apnoea, paralysis and coma.

Treatment involves cessation of administration, intravenous fluids and standard resuscitation with airway protection, intubation, ventilation and inotropic support if required. There is no antidote.

Allergic reactions to local anaesthetics are extremely uncommon.

7. Bier's block

What is a Bier's block and how is it applied?

Bier's block is a form of intravenous regional anaesthesia usually of the upper limb, established by direct intravenous administration of local anaesthetic into a limb, previously isolated from the systemic circulation by a tourniquet. It is used as a regional block, and is useful for upper limb procedures, e.g. reduction of Colles' fracture, removal of foreign body.

First, intravenous access is established in both arms, on the affected side for administration of the block, and on the unaffected side for rapid intravenous access in case of resuscitation requirements. Then the limb is exsanguinated, the tourniquet is applied and 20-40ml of prilocaine injected below the cuff intravenously.

What are the dangers and complications?

The main danger is systemic toxicity due to cuff failure or releasing the cuff too early (it takes 30 minutes for the local anaesthetic to bind in the tissues, preventing systemic spread). To prevent this, a double cuff is employed as a safeguard. This has the additional advantage that the lower cuff can be inflated over anaesthetised skin to reduce pain under the cuff. Prilocaine is the local anaesthetic of choice as it is less cardiotoxic, and has a shorter half-life. Bupivacaine is contraindicated as it is too toxic. Other complications can be caused by the tourniquet (see section 2.7.12).

8. Transfer of the anaesthetised patient

The patient is on a trolley in the anaesthetic room. Describe the stages in transfer of the patient to the operating table

When the patient is ready for transfer, all lines, drips, catheters and electronic monitoring are either temporarily disconnected or placed on or adjacent to the patient on the canvas draw sheet. After ensuring the patient is well oxygenated the airway is disconnected from the anaesthetic machine, the brakes are taken off the trolley with the sides up and the trolley is wheeled into theatre. The trolley is placed alongside the operating table, brakes reapplied and airway connected. The trolley sides are lowered and a plastic slide is positioned from the operating table side of the patient, under the canvas draw sheet, to bridge the gap between the trolley and the table. On the anaesthetist's instructions the patient is slid across before the plastic slide is removed from the trolley side of the patient. All lines and monitoring are then reconnected and appropriately placed.

What areas have to be especially cared for during the transfer of an anaesthetised patient?

◆ Airway - avoid dislodgement of the endotracheal tube or laryngeal mask.
◆ Cervical spine - especially in the elderly, or if there is a suspicion of instability.
◆ Monitoring/drips/catheters.
◆ Limbs - can fall between the trolley and table, causing nerve injuries, bruising, dislocations, etc.

9. Care of the anaesthetised patient

What special precautions have to be taken to ensure an anaesthetised patient comes to no harm whilst undergoing procedures in the operating theatre?

◆ Airway - must stay connected and be monitored at all times. Most modern ventilators have alarms to prevent inadvertent disconnection.

2.6.8

2.6.9

- Eyes - are usually taped shut, often with eye pads and lubricant.
- Hair - if long should be in a theatre cap to prevent tangling with table/lines/monitoring, etc.
- Cervical spine - should be neutrally placed with collar and head restraints if unstable.
- Arms - should be secured, usually either at the patient's side or on an arm board to prevent flailing.
- Skin - should not be in contact with metal to prevent diathermy short circuit burns.
- Pressure areas - especially heels, buttocks, shoulders and the back of the head. Padding or heel protectors should be considered for longer operations.
- Diathermy plate - should be appropriately placed where it will not get wet and will not be over bony prominences, metal prostheses, or near pacemakers or monitoring equipment. Application is best over a large even surface, to prevent burns.
- Thermoregulation - the patient should be kept warm with drapes, or for long operations have a warming mattress or plastic warm air cover to prevent cold injury. If large volumes of rapidly-infused intravenous fluids are given they should be administered through a fluid warming device.
- Nerve injury - some nerves are particularly susceptible to injury on the operating table, e.g. ulnar nerve by direct pressure from arm supports, peroneal nerve in lithotomy position, sural nerve with short saphenous varicose vein surgery, accessory nerve with operations in the posterior triangle of the neck.
- Deep venous thrombosis prophylaxis - stockings, pneumatic calf compression devices (see section 1.3.5).

Chapter 7

Principles of surgery

1. Peripheral lines

Describe the principles of safe peripheral venous cannulation

Peripheral venous access is required for introducing intravenous fluids or drugs, or taking blood samples. The most commonly used veins are large forearm veins, (cephalic, basilic, median antecubital veins) and the hand veins. Other sites include femoral vein, external jugular vein, long saphenous vein at the ankle, and scalp veins in neonates. Local anaesthesia can be administered at the site where the cannula is to be placed, to reduce pain on insertion.

A cannula is introduced after placing a tourniquet proximal to the site of insertion to cause venous engorgement, and the skin is cleaned at the chosen site. The cannula is then introduced on an obturator needle and the needle withdrawn, leaving the plastic catheter in place. The cap is then placed on the device to prevent bleeding, and the device secured with adhesive tape.

2.7.1

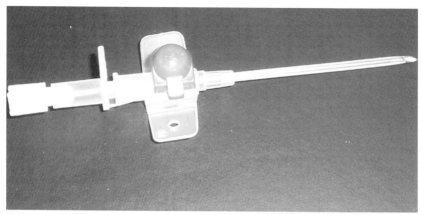

Figure 1. Peripheral cannula (Venflon™).

What are the complications of peripheral venous cannulation?

Bleeding, subcutaneous haematoma, extravasion of infused fluid, thrombophlebitis, infection, artery or nerve damage, e.g. brachial artery or median nerve in the antecubital fossa.

What are the alternatives to peripheral venous cannulation?

In severely shocked patients the peripheral veins may be collapsed precluding cannulation. In patients having had chemotherapy or IV drug abusers, the peripheral veins may be thrombosed. Alternative routes of IV access include central line placement (see section 2.7.2) or surgical venous cut down, where venous access is acquired by direct incision over the vein and open surgical exposure (usually the long saphenous vein at the ankle). In children, fluids can be rapidly infused via the intra-osseous route, usually via the upper tibia.

2. Central lines

How is a central venous pressure catheter inserted?

The patient is placed in the head-down position to prevent air embolism and distend the veins. After scrubbing, and donning sterile gown and gloves, the skin is prepared over the subclavian or internal jugular vein. Traditionally, the vein is located by palpation or by anatomical landmarks. The vein can also be located by ultrasound guidance. A long needle is advanced towards the vein until venous blood can be withdrawn. A guidewire is then threaded down the needle (Seldinger technique), and the needle withdrawn. A dilator is then passed down the guidewire followed by the catheter, which is then advanced over the wire until correctly positioned, and the wire withdrawn. The catheter is secured, usually with a stitch and a check X-ray is performed to ensure correct positioning, and to exclude accidental pneumothorax or haemothorax.

2.7.2

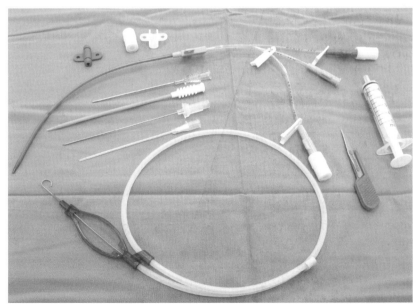

Figure 2. Central line.

What are the complications of central venous catheter placement?

◆ Immediate: incorrect placement, pneumothorax, air embolism, accidental arterial puncture, lost guidewire, haemothorax, arrhythmias, cardiac perforation.
◆ Delayed: line sepsis, abscess, false aneurysm, nerve injury (brachial plexus, phrenic), thoracic duct injury, arteriovenous fistula.

3. Arterial lines

What is an arterial line?

An arterial line is a plastic cannula, placed in an artery to gain access to the arterial lumen for arterial blood sampling and/or pressure measurement. The most commonly placed arterial line is a radial artery line at the wrist, although femoral artery lines and brachial lines are also available.

How are arterial lines used?

The cannula is connected via a three-way tap to a pressure transducer, so real time arterial blood pressure can be monitored. This is essential for major vascular, cardiac and neurosurgical procedures. Arterial lines are also used for obtaining arterial blood samples for blood gas analysis.

What are the complications of arterial lines?

◆ Immediate: displacement leading to bleeding or haematoma.
◆ Early: distal embolisation, arterial spasm causing distal ischaemia, infection, cannula disruption with retained intra-arterial foreign body.
◆ Late: false aneurysm, arterial damage causing distal ischaemia, arteriovenous fistula.

Arterial lines should be clearly labelled, as accidental injection of intravenous drugs can cause severe distal tissue injury.

4. Catheters

What is a catheter?

A catheter is a tube used to gain access into organs or vessels of the body to introduce or drain fluids, or take samples.

2.7.4

Give some examples of commonly used catheters

◆ Peripheral venous catheterisation (or cannulation) - a Venflon™ is introduced into a peripheral vein for giving intravenous fluids or drugs, or taking blood samples (see section 2.7.1).

◆ Central venous catheterisation (or cannulation) - a central venous catheter is introduced into the subclavian or internal jugular vein. It is used for introducing intravenous fluids or drugs, intravenous feeding, withdrawing blood samples or measuring central venous pressure (see section 2.7.2).

◆ Urinary catheter (or Foley catheter) - is introduced into the bladder either via the urethra (urethral catheter), or suprapubically (suprapubic catheter) through the anterior abdominal wall. It is used

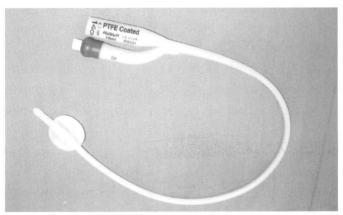

Figure 3. Foley catheter.

for draining urine from the bladder (or measuring urine output). It has a balloon to prevent accidental displacement.

◆ Nasogastric tube - is a catheter introduced via the nose into the stomach (or jejunum - nasojejunal tube). It is used for gastric drainage after major abdominal surgery, or for enteral feeding.

◆ Fogarty catheter - is a special sort of catheter with a balloon to withdraw blood clots from occluded blood vessels.

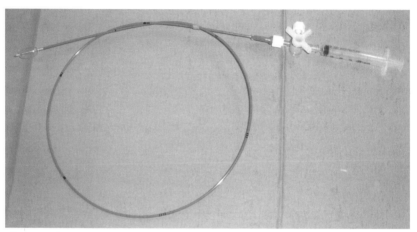

Figure 4. Fogarty catheter.

◆ Cardiac catheter - is the name given to the tube introduced via an artery (usually femoral) and advanced into the coronary ostea for coronary angiography, or angioplasty and stenting.

What are the complications of catheters?

Blockage, dislodgement, bleeding, malpositioning, infection, removal problems, e.g. catheters may become stuck or break.

5. Drains

What are surgical drains?

A means by which fluid is moved either between a real, potential or pathological space and the external environment or between one compartment or cavity and another. Surgical drains are used primarily to remove fluids, liquid or gas, and for the closure of 'dead' space through the apposition of tissues from a suction effect.

Classify surgical drains

Surgical drains are classified as open or closed systems.

An open drain has open ends, such as a corrugated or Penrose drain. The ribbon gauze or wicks in otitis externa or a peri-anal abscess are types of open drains.

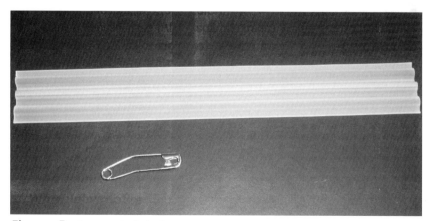

Figure 5. Corrugated drain.

Closed drains have a closed end, such as the Jackson-Pruitt or Redivac™ drains, which are tubes attached to suction bottles. Closed systems can be further classified as those with or without suction, i.e. relying on gravity alone. Chest drains are described in section 3.10.12.

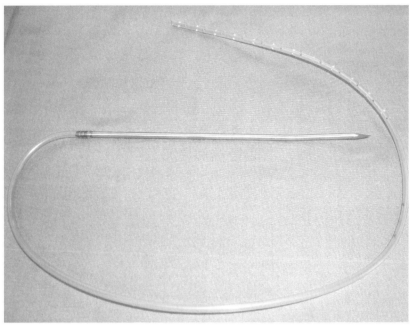

Figure 6. Suction drain.

What are the complications of surgical drains?

◆ Blockage.
◆ Dislodgement.
◆ Bleeding - drains may erode into blood vessels.
◆ Malpositioning.
◆ Siphoning, e.g. a chest drain placed above chest height may cause reintroduction of drained fluids into the chest cavity.
◆ Infection.
◆ Removal problems, e.g. drains may adhere to tissues and become stuck or break, or may be inadvertently sutured deep in the wound requiring open retrieval.

6. Sutures

How would you classify suture materials?

◆ Absorbable v non-absorbable.
◆ Braided v monofilament.
◆ Synthetic v natural.

Examples of the different types of sutures are as follows:

◆ Prolene (polypropylene) is a non-absorbable, synthetic monofilament. It is widely used for wound closure, vascular anastomosis, etc.
◆ Polyglactic acid (vicryl) is a braided, absorbable, synthetic suture. It is generally used for tissue approximation and as a ligature.
◆ Polydioxanone sulphate (PDS) is an absorbable, synthetic monofilament. It is used for internal tissue approximation and has a longer half life than vicryl.
◆ Silk is a non-absorbable, braided, natural suture. It is no longer widely used, but is occasionally used to secure drains.
◆ Catgut is an absorbable, natural suture. It is no longer widely used.

Generally, monofilament sutures cause less tissue reaction. Braided sutures tie easily but cause more tissue reaction and possibly promote infections and 'stitch abscesses'. Absorbable sutures always cause a tissue reaction by definition as they are broken down by tissue enzymes. Non-absorbable sutures have the obvious advantage that they are a permanent tissue support, but the disadvantage, like any foreign body, is that they may provoke a tissue reaction and are a potential infection risk.

Explain how sutures are sized

Many years ago the sutures used were much larger than they are now and the smallest available was gauge 1. As smaller sutures were developed it became necessary to go backwards in gauge system. So the next smallest was 0 and then 00, 000 and so on. 00 is expressed as 2/0 and 000 as 3/0. The smallest available suture now is 10/0.

What information is available to the surgeon on a suture packet?

Suture material trade name and generic name, description (e.g. braided or coated), suture size, length of suture, needle type and number of needles, company code number, expiration date and manufacturer's name.

7. Needles and blades

What are the types of suture needle and what are their main uses?

Suture needles differ in the type of cutting edge and body shape. Cutting types include tapered, conventional cutting, reverse cutting and a blunt tip. Tapered needles are usually used for closing delicate tissue such as a vascular anastomosis or intestinal mucosa, as they are less traumatic. Conventional cutting needles are used for tougher tissues such as skin. Reverse cutting needles were designed to cut tissues easily and are used for very tough tissues or when minimal tissue reaction is required, such as in ophthalmic surgery. Blunt needles were specially designed for liver and kidney surgery. The needles are available in straight or curved shapes in almost any length. Curved needles include ¼, 3/8, 5/8, ½ circle, as well as a 'j' shape and half curved, which is a straight needle with a curve at the cutting end.

Describe the main features of three most commonly used scalpel blades

The number 10 blade is a large knife blade used for large incisions on the body or scalp. It is usually held like a steak knife at 30° to the surface. The belly of the blade is the cutting edge not the tip.

The number 15 blade is a smaller knife used for more delicate surgery such as facial incisions. It is held in a pencil grip at 45° to the surface.

The number 11 blade is a triangular pointed blade. It is used for making puncture wounds using the tip of the blade, such as incising an abscess or inserting a drain or trocar.

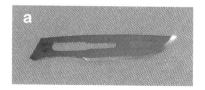
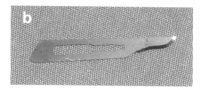
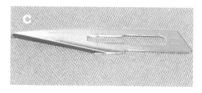

Figure 7. Scalpel blades, numbers: a) 10, b) 15, c) 11.

8. Diathermy

How does surgical diathermy work?

Diathermy is the generation of heat by the passage of high frequency alternating current. It is used in surgery to cut tissues and to control bleeding through coagulation. The patient is not electrocuted in spite of the high voltage due to the very high frequency of the current. Normal domestic alternating current is at 60Hz; the frequencies used for diathermy are in the region of 0.5 to 1.5MHz. The effect of diathermy depends on the current density and waveform. Denser current produces more heat and more tissue destruction. Damped waveforms at the lower end of the frequency range (0.4MHz) produce coagulation whilst sine waveforms at 1 to 1.5MHz produce cutting. Blended waveforms can produce cutting and coagulation.

2.7.8

What are the types of diathermy?

There are two types of diathermy in use: monopolar and bipolar.

Monopolar or unipolar diathermy consists of a circuit which runs from the electrode, which is in the surgeon's hand (the active part), through the patient's tissues to the electrode plate which is adherent to a large flat, dry surface of the patient's skin.

Bipolar diathermy involves the current running only between tissue held between the tips of the forceps and is used for coagulation, especially when there is a contraindication to monopolar diathermy, such as patients with pacemakers or when there is a risk of current concentration, e.g. in digit surgery.

What are the dangers of diathermy use?

◆ Accidental activation causing burns.
◆ Monopolar diathermy can cause unnecessary tissue damage if there is a long uninsulated electrode end and the surgeon is working in a confined space.
◆ Fires and explosions, especially with flammable, alcohol-based skin preparations and oxygen.
◆ Current concentration, for example, if the return electrode is not properly attached to the patient then heat will be generated and a burn will occur. Similarly, in surgery to the fingers or penis, current concentration can cause significant tissue damage.
◆ In laparoscopic surgery, capacitance coupling can cause tissue damage and burning.
◆ In patients with pacemakers and implanted defibrillators, there is a danger that the current could cause interruption or stimulation, especially if the surgery electrode and plate electrode are on opposite sides of the heart.
◆ The electrode tips remain hot after use and may cause unintended tissue damage.

9. Retractors

What is a surgical retractor and what are the principles of retraction?

A retractor is an instrument used to move tissues aside to facilitate views of the area to be operated on. Retraction is performed by gentle traction or counter-traction, usually on the skin and subcutaneous tissues of an incision. Retraction needs to be firm enough to give adequate exposure, but not so violent as to cause tissue damage by pressure necrosis, ischaemia or skin or tissue tearing.

What types of retractor do you know and what are their uses?

♦ Simple retraction - can be performed with the hand or fingers, or with a hand-held retractor, e.g. Langenbeck, Kelly, Deaver. These are simply pulled back against the wound edge.

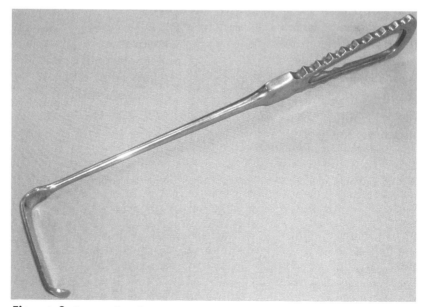

Figure 8. Langenbeck retractor.

- ◆ Tape or sling retraction - tapes or slings can be passed around vessels, nerves or tendons to gently pull them aside to expose underlying structures.
- ◆ Self-retaining retractors - have a hinge and ratchet, so they pull back both sides of a wound and maintain their position without being held, e.g. Travers self-retainer, Parkes anal retractor, Golligher retractor.

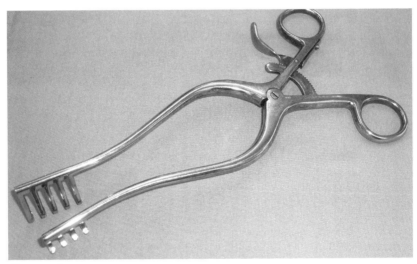

Figure 9. Self-retaining retractor.

- ◆ Fixed retraction devices - are complex systems of retractors, usually on rings or bars, which work by counter-traction at the sides of large wounds, and are fixed to the operating table sides or to a bar across the table, e.g. Omnitract®.

10. Forceps

Classify forceps

Forceps are used to grasp, retract or stabilise tissue. They are broadly classified as non-toothed or toothed.

2.7.10

Explain their uses

Non-toothed forceps are generally used for the gentle handling of fragile tissue, such as blood vessels, as they are less traumatic, e.g. De Bakey forceps.

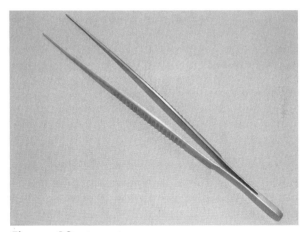

Figure 10. Tissue forceps.

Toothed forceps provide more grip, but are more traumatic, e.g. Gillies forceps.

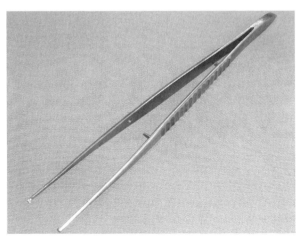

Figure 11. Gillies forceps.

Heavy duty multiple toothed forceps, e.g. Adson forceps, are used for grasping tough tissue or when more force is required. Dental forceps are specialised instruments for the removal of teeth.

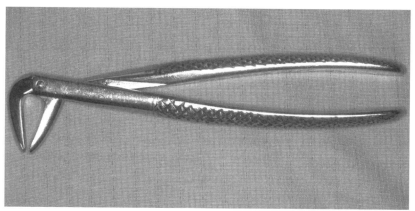

Figure 12. Dental forceps.

11. Suction and theatre waste

How does a theatre suction system work?

The principle of theatre suction is to keep the operating field free from excess fluid, to facilitate a good view for the surgeon. The non-disposable portions of the suction system, should not get exposed to body fluids, and the waste fluids need to be safely disposed of.

The usual system consists of an electrically driven vacuum pump device, that creates a vacuum in a disposable reservoir, via a non-return valve, to prevent the vacuum pump coming into contact with body fluids. The reservoir is connected via a filter to the suction tubing, which is plugged into the surgeon's hand-held sucker. The surgeon's end of the suction tubing remains sterile. The vacuum pump is adjustable to create different forces of suction for different operations.

2.7.11

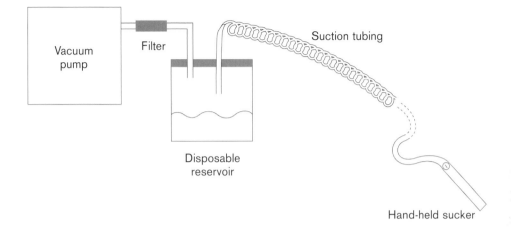

Figure 13. Theatre suction system.

What happens to the sucked up fluid?

When the reservoir is full a solidifying pellet is added so the contents of the reservoir are turned to a solid gel, for safe disposal. The whole sealed reservoir cylinder can then be placed in the clinical waste disposal bin for incineration.

What types of sucker do you know?

♦   Yankauer sucker - a disposable plastic general purpose sucker for evacuation of normal blood and body fluids. The tip is offset to allow accurate placement for suction in deep wounds or in the airway.

♦   Pool-guarded sucker - a reusable metal sucker with a guard with holes to prevent solid tissue and organs adhering to the sucker.

♦   Fine vascular sucker - for extra sensitive areas.

♦   Frazer fenestrated suction - gentle guarded suction for ENT operations.

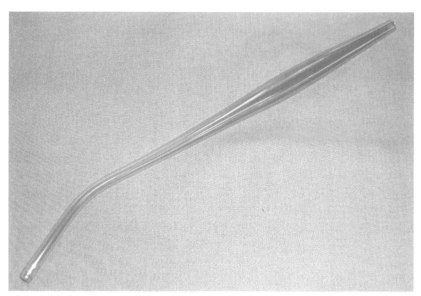

Figure 14. Yankauer sucker.

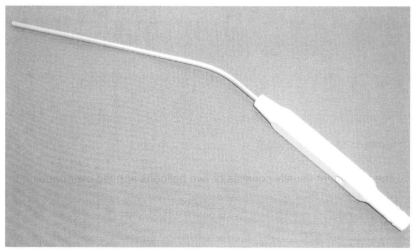

Figure 15. Fine suction.

What are the categories of theatre waste?

This is now almost universal in hospitals:

◆ Yellow bag - contaminated theatre waste, dressings, etc. - for incineration.
◆ Yellow box (sharps box/bucket) - has a guarded lid. For all sharps, contaminated or otherwise - for incineration.
◆ Red/orange bag - used for linen, contaminated or otherwise. The sealed bag is put unopened in the laundry where the hot wash dissolves the alginate bag releasing the contents. The clean linen is then folded and packed for sterilisation (see section 2.5.7).
◆ Black bag - non-clinical waste, paper, etc. - for conventional disposal.

12. Tourniquets

What is a tourniquet and when should it be used?

A tourniquet is a device placed around a limb or digit, to prevent bleeding or isolate perfusion:

◆ Simple tourniquet - usually an elastic strip, bandage or cuff, e.g. elastic tourniquet for phlebotomy, rubber tourniquet to prevent bleeding during ingrowing toenail surgery.
◆ Limb tourniquet - used to prevent bleeding in limb surgery, or isolate the limb, e.g. for Bier's block (see section 2.6.7).

Method of application:

The tourniquet usually consists of two balloons applied over padding to prevent pressure injury around the limb. The balloons are pneumatically inflated to above systolic pressure to prevent arterial and venous bleeding during limb surgery:

◆ Upper limb - inflate to approximately 50mm Hg over systolic.
◆ Lower limb - inflate to approximately 100mm Hg over systolic.

2.7.12

Lower pressures are needed for children. Note the time of application. The cuff should be deflated after two hours to prevent ischaemic injury. A tourniquet should not be used as a first aid measure to stop bleeding (except in battlefield injuries).

What are the complications of tourniquets?

◆   Pressure necrosis from an overtight tourniquet or insufficient padding.
◆   Ischaemic necrosis from prolonged application.
◆   Distal ischaemia from arterial thrombosis.
◆   DVT or superficial venous thrombosis.
◆   Skin, muscle or joint damage due to lack of care on application or structures getting caught in the tourniquet, e.g. genitalia with a thigh tourniquet.
◆   Haemorrhage following release.
◆   Metabolic disturbances following release after prolonged application, e.g. lactic acidosis, hyperkalaemia.

13. Lasers

What is a laser and how does it work?

LASER (Light Amplification by Stimulated Emission of Radiation).

Lasers produce light by high voltage stimulation of a medium, producing photons which are then bounced around inside the medium producing more photons until all the photons in phase are released through a narrow aperture producing a beam of intensely bright light. This is capable of cutting or burning tissue, and causing coagulation. The beam can be introduced through narrow apertures, for example, down laparoscopes, and fine beams are capable of precise cutting or coagulation with minimal damage to surrounding tissues.

2.7.13

What are their applications?

- Argon beam laser - eye surgery, endoscopic surgery.
- CO_2 laser - ENT, laparoscopic or cervical ablation surgery.
- ND:YAG laser - coagulation of bleeding vessels, endoscopic and laparoscopic surgery.

What are their complications?

- Damage to adjacent structures.
- Burns (to patient or surgeon).
- Eye damage (to patient or surgeon).
- Fire risk.

Chapter 8

Basic surgical techniques

1. Surgical wounds

Define wound, laceration, abrasion, incision and dissection

◆ A wound is a break in the skin or an organ as a result of surgery or trauma.
◆ A laceration is a cut, tear or ragged opening in tissues or skin caused by trauma.
◆ An abrasion is traumatic removal of superficial skin.
◆ An incision is a sharp cut into tissues.
◆ Dissection is the purposeful separation of tissues. It may be sharp or blunt.

What are the means by which a surgeon can cut tissue?

Tissues can be cut by scalpel, scissors, cutting diathermy (see section 2.7.8) or laser (see section 2.7.13). The tissues may be separated by sharp or blunt dissection. Surgical stapling devices cut and may staple the edges to join or anastomose tissues or hollow viscera (see section 2.8.2). The Harmonic Scalpel™ uses ultrasonic frequencies to cut and synchronously coagulate tissues.

2.8.1

What is primary wound closure?

The wound is sutured closed immediately, otherwise known as healing by primary intention. It causes minimal scarring and is considered the ideal means of wound closure.

What is secondary closure?

Secondary closure is when a wound is left open and heals without suturing by a combination of granulation, contraction and eventual epithelialisation over a course of weeks. It causes more scarring but in cases of dirty, contaminated wounds after debridement, it may be the optimal means of wound healing. Secondary revision surgery, when scars are excised and closed primarily, may be considered at a later date.

Delayed primary closure is when a wound is sutured closed some three to five days after incision. This is sometimes used for infected wounds.

What are the key features of a wound that lead to ideal healing?

Local factors:

The scar should be within or parallel to a relaxed skin crease. The wound should have accurate skin approximation and freedom from infection and haematoma. Previous radiotherapy, rough tissue handling and poor blood supply may delay healing.

Systemic factors:

General factors which are important in healing include sepsis, malignancy, anaemia, hypoxia, diabetes, steroids and other immunocompromise, general poor blood supply, such as heart failure, and malnutrition, especially protein, zinc and vitamins A and C.

2. Surgical stitches

What types of surgical stitch do you know?

◆ Simple interrupted - used for simple wound or laceration closure. Interrupted sutures are usually non-absorbable and need to be removed.

2.8.2

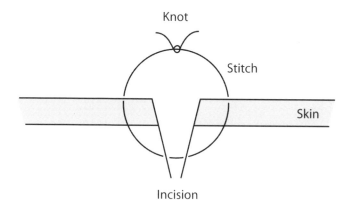

Figure 1. Simple stitch.

◆ Interrupted mattress - these stitches pierce the tissue twice at each side of the wound, to provide extra strength, and are used for wounds under tension or with the potential for poor healing. They are usually non-absorbable and need to be removed.

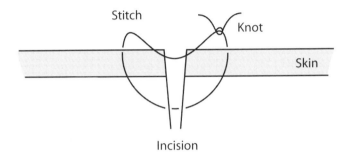

Figure 2. Interrupted mattress stitch.

◆ Continuous suture - this single over-and-over stitch is used for apposing deeper tissues, e.g. abdominal wall closure (see section 2.8.4). It may be absorbable or non-absorbable, but does not need to be removed.
◆ Continuous mattress - this stitch is occasionally used for long skin wounds.
◆ Subcuticular suture - this is a skin closure stitch where the stitch is placed under the skin, immediately adjacent to the wound. It leaves clean linear scars and is usually absorbable so it does not need to be removed.

What alternatives to stitches are there for tissue approximation?

◆ Steristrips™ or surgical tape - for small skin incisions.
◆ Staples - these are small metal clips, usually used for long clean incisions. They need to be removed by a clip remover.
◆ Glue:
  ● cyanoacrylate (tissue glue, Dermabond™) is often used for epidermal wound edge approximation in small clean wounds, particularly in children in the Accident and Emergency Department. This technique may reduce scarring;
  ● fibrin glue (Tisseel™) can be used for deep wounds (e.g. in neurosurgery for dural tears), or for large raw exposed areas (e.g. in hepatobiliary surgery for haemostasis following liver resection).
◆ Surgical stapling devices - circular or linear staplers cut and staple tissue to close or join viscera. They are used for bowel anastomosis, or in thoracic surgery for lung resection.

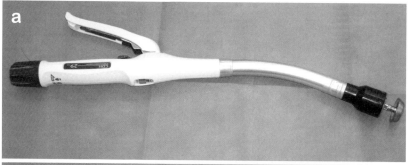

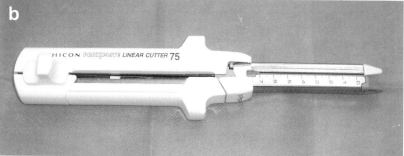

Figure 3. Surgical stapling devices. a) Circular stapler. b) Linear stapler.

3. Abdominal incisions

How do you open an abdomen?

The patient is usually supine on the operating table under general anaesthetic, intubated, ventilated and paralysed. Different abdominal operations are performed through different incisions. The best access to the abdominal cavity is through a mid-line incision. This is performed by first using a scalpel to incise the skin along the mid-line, skirting the umbilicus. The incision is deepened through the superficial fascia and fat using a scalpel, or cutting diathermy blade. Small blood vessels are coagulated by diathermy, or ligated. When the muscle layers are reached, the linea alba (mid-line) is incised longitudinally with a scalpel, then cut with strong scissors between the rectus muscles. The peritoneum is picked up with two clips, and pinched to ensure no abdominal viscera are stuck to it. It is incised with a scalpel and then divided superiorly and inferiorly with scissors to complete the abdominal incision.

What sort of abdominal incisions do you know?

- ◆ A Lanz.
- ◆ B Grid iron.
- ◆ C Rutherford-Morrison.
- ◆ D Pfannenstiel.
- ◆ E Kocher.
- ◆ F Roof top.
- ◆ G Paramedian.
- ◆ H Supra-umbilical
- ◆ I Transverse.
- ◆ J Mid-line.

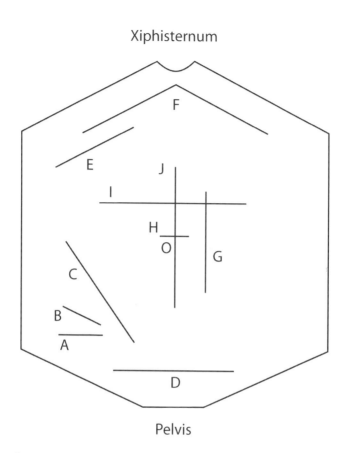

Figure 4. Abdominal incisions.

4. Abdominal wall closure

What are the principles of abdominal wall closure?

Mid-line abdominal incisions are best closed by a mass closure technique. This incorporates all the layers of the abdominal wall, except the skin (peritoneum, posterior and anterior rectus sheath, rectus muscle and some superficial fascia), into the closure. Continuous sutures for mass closure are used with 0 or 1.0 nylon or PDS (polydioxanone

2.8.4

sulphate). Suture bites should be placed 1cm apart and 2cm from the wound edge. The sutures should be pulled tightly enough to appose the sides of the wound, but not so tight as to strangulate the muscles. It is estimated that adequate closure requires sufficient suture to reach four times the length of the wound incision (Jenkins law).

The skin is then apposed with subcuticular sutures, interrupted mattress sutures or skin clips (see section 2.8.2).

What are the consequences of poor abdominal wall closure?

♦ Wound infection.
♦ Wound dehiscence.
♦ Burst abdomen.
♦ Late incisional hernia.

5. Thoracotomy

What are the principles of thoracotomy?

A thoracotomy is an incision into the thoracic (chest) cavity. It can be attained by median sternotomy (for access to the heart and great vessels, hila of the lungs, thymus and retrosternal thyroid), through a left posterolateral thoracotomy (for access to the left lung, aorta, oesophagus, left ventricle), or a right posterolateral thoracotomy (for access to the right lung, right ventricle and oesophagus).

A posterolateral thoracotomy is achieved by incision through skin, chest wall muscles and intercostal muscles, running the incision immediately above the rib to avoid damage to the neurovascular bundle. The ribs are carefully pulled apart using a ratcheted 'rib spreader' retractor. Special care must be taken in retracting delicate lung tissue to expose underlying structures. If necessary, the lungs can be partially deflated using one lung ventilation, a special anaesthetic technique.

2.8.5

A posterolateral thoracotomy is closed by re-apposing ribs and muscle with non-absorbable suture, e.g. nylon or with wire suture. A chest drain with underwater sealed drainage is left in the pleural cavity to prevent a pneumothorax/haemothorax (see section 3.10.12).

A median sternotomy is achieved by a midline incision through skin, and powersaw midline division of the sternum. Care is needed due to the proximity of the heart and great vessels. Closure is usually by interrupted wire suture re-apposition.

What are the complications of thoracotomy?

Lung/heart/vessel injury, haemothorax, pneumothorax, diaphragmatic injury, nerve injury (vagus, phrenic, sympathetic nerves), post-thoracotomy neuralgia, rib fracture and non-union, sternal non-union, and infection (pneumonia, empyema, mediastinitis).

6. Anastomosis

What is an anastomosis?

An anastomosis is the process by which two or more hollow viscera, organs or vessels are joined to allow transit between their lumina.

What are the principles of an anastomosis?

Safe anastomosis requires the join to be tension-free, with accurate apposition of the walls and good size approximation of the lumina. Bowel and genitourinary anastomoses require a good blood supply to the ends and the join should have no holes or leaks.

Failure of an anastomosis can be due to local or general factors:

◆ Local factors: for example, poor surgical technique, inadequate mobilisation of ends leading to tension, and poor blood supply.
◆ General factors: for example, old age, malnutrition, malignancy, sepsis.

How are anastomoses formed?

◆ Sutures - interrupted or continuous, absorbable or non-absorbable (see section 2.8.2).
◆ Staples - used in some gastrointestinal anastomoses.
◆ Glue - for some vessel and neural anastomoses.

7. Biopsy

What is a biopsy?

Biopsy is retrieval of tissue, or part of an organ, for pathological evaluation, e.g. histology, cytology, microbiology. It can be used to establish a tissue diagnosis, diagnose malignancy or extent of spread, and retrieve samples for microbiological examination.

What techniques of biopsy are available to a surgeon?

◆ Excisional biopsy - where a whole lesion is excised to establish a histological diagnosis, e.g. excision of basal cell carcinoma.
◆ Incisional biopsy - part of a lesion is excised to obtain histology. It is used for lesions which are too big or fixed for complete excision, or where complete excision may not be required. It may be performed laparoscopically or by open incision.
◆ Endoscopic biopsy - retrieved by endoscopy, e.g. gastrointestinal tract, bladder, airways, uterus. The advantage is that it may avoid open surgery, but it can cause bleeding and perforation, and as small samples are taken it is possible that the malignant area may be missed.
◆ Core biopsy - performed using a penetrating circular cutting instrument (e.g. Trucut®) for breast, liver or lymph node biopsy. This technique has the advantage that it is relatively simple, in some cases can be performed in an outpatient setting and can be repeated several times if insufficient tissue is obtained. However, even when performed under ultrasound guidance it can damage neighbouring structures, such as blood vessels, nerves and the lungs, and there may be problematic bleeding. It is also quite uncomfortable.

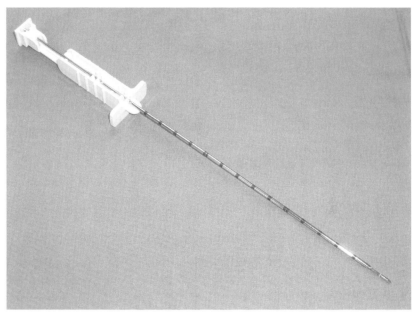

Figure 5. Trucut® biopsy device.

◆ Frozen section - a special sort of biopsy where fresh tissue is sent for immediate histological assessment during an operation, to obtain rapid tissue diagnosis and aid peri-operative decision-making, e.g. frozen section of thyroid tissue to establish malignancy, allowing a decision to proceed to either a thyroid lobectomy or a total thyroidectomy, while the patient is still anaesthetised.

◆ Cytology - a simple sort of biopsy where cells are retrieved and sent for cytological analysis to aid diagnosis, for example:

  • fine needle aspiration cytology - a fine bore needle is inserted into a lesion, aspirating cells to produce a smear on a slide for cytological examination;

  • brush cytology - cells are retrieved by brushing a small brush against a lesion, often used endoscopically.

The advantages are that it is simple, cheap, minimally invasive and easily repeatable. The disadvantages include obtaining cytological but not architectural histology, insufficient samples, bleeding and the potential for spread of malignant cells.

8. Abscess

What is an abscess?

An abscess is a localised collection of pus. It is part of the body's normal response to infection and consists of neutrophils, bacteria, dead cells and other debris. Abscesses usually present as red, hot, tender fluctuant swellings, often with a head or 'pointing' area on the skin. Deep abscesses are more difficult to diagnose. Ultrasound or needle aspiration can be used to aid diagnosis.

How is it treated?

Left alone, many abscesses will drain spontaneously. Otherwise, abscesses should be surgically drained. Superficial abscesses can be lanced or drained under local anaesthetic. Deep abscesses require general anaesthetic. Pus is sent for microbiological examination, culture and sensitivities. The abscess cavity is thoroughly lavaged and gently packed, usually with a gauze wick. The packing is changed daily until the cavity closes.

Complications of abscess drainage include recurrence, inadequate drainage (especially loculated abscesses), persistent cellulitis requiring antibiotics, or damage to other structures during drainage, e.g. accessory nerve in neck abscesses.

9. Minimal access surgery

What is minimal access surgery?

Minimal access surgery is performed through incisions, or via orifices smaller than and/or remote from that required for conventional surgery, for example:

♦   General surgery - laparoscopic cholecystectomy, laparoscopic appendicectomy.

- Colorectal - laparoscopic hemicolectomy, laparoscopic-assisted anterior resection.
- Orthopaedics - arthroscopy.
- Urology - cystoscopy, transurethral resection of the prostate, laparoscopic nephrectomy.
- Vascular - transluminal angioplasty, endovascular aneurysm repair.
- Gynaecology - laparoscopic sterilisation, laparoscopic oophorectomy.
- Thoracic - thoracoscopic sympathectomy, thoracoscopic lobectomy.

What are the advantages and disadvantages of minimal access surgery?

- Advantages: smaller wounds, less painful, less wound complications, shorter hospital stay, quick return to normal activities.
- Disadvantages: equipment can be expensive, complications due to damage to adjacent structures, takes longer, may be difficult to control bleeding, sometimes impossible due to adhesions from previous surgery.

10. Day-case surgery

What is day surgery?

Day surgery is the planned admission of a patient for a surgical procedure with discharge the same day. Although it includes local and general anaesthesia it excludes procedures which are performed in an outpatient setting, such as tooth removal, colposcopy and some dermatological procedures. Day surgery includes 23-hour-stay surgery, where the patient has the procedure, and is discharged early the next morning, so the bed is available for another patient.

2.8.10

What are the advantages and disadvantages?

The advantages are a shorter hospital stay causing less disruption to patients' lives and this may have a psychological benefit, especially for children. There is a reduced risk of acquiring nosocomial infections and less chance of having the operation cancelled at the last minute, as emergency operating is less likely to intrude on a day surgery list.

The potential disadvantages are that the patient may be discharged home before they feel ready or they may require unplanned admission in the event of complications or prolonged recovery.

What are the criteria for day surgery?

Safe day-case surgery requires three things: the right patient having the right operation in the right environment.

The patient criteria include physical health and social factors. They should generally be in category ASA 1 or 2, although in recent years patients in category ASA 3 have been included if their disease is well controlled (see section 1.3.1). Children should be ASA 1 or 2. The Body Mass Index has been important in the past with a ceiling of 35, although in many units now, this upper limit has been removed.

Social factors are also important. The patient should live within approximately one hour's drive of the hospital and there must be a responsible adult to accompany the patient home, look after the patient at home after the operation and if necessary return the patient to hospital. There must be a telephone at home.

The type of operation is important. It should be a relatively quick procedure (under one hour) and have a low incidence of complications. Local anaesthetic procedures are ideal. If the procedure is such that the patient requires postoperative opiate analgesia and subsequently a prolonged recovery, then the procedure is not suitable for day-case surgery.

The day unit should have facilities for admission if required. It should be set up to screen the patients pre-operatively to ensure the criteria are met. This is usually nurse-run with access to a dedicated anaesthetist.

Section 3

Postoperative care and complications

Chapter 9

Recovery and immediate postoperative care

1. Recovery

What is a theatre recovery area?

The theatre recovery area or post-anaesthetic care unit (PACU) is a zone for postoperative patients who require a period of physiological stabilisation. It is staffed by specialist nurses and has monitoring facilities similar to an intensive care unit. It is located within the theatre suite to reduce the potentially dangerous transit time between the operating room and the ward. It is also essential to have anaesthetic and surgical staff close at hand in the event that additional help is required in the PACU or if the patient needs to return to theatre urgently.

What is the minimum monitoring required for immediate post-procedural care (recovery)?

This depends on the nature of the surgery and the anaesthetic performed. Minor surgery under local anaesthetic requires very little immediate post-procedural care. Minimum monitoring following general anaesthesia usually requires pulse rate and blood pressure monitoring,

3.9.1

respiratory rate monitoring, an ECG trace, pulse oximetry and temperature measurement.

What are the most common postoperative complications encountered in the recovery department?

◆ Respiratory - hypoventilation, hypoxaemia, airway obstruction.
◆ Cardiovascular - hypertension, hypotension, arrhythmias, myocardial ischaemia.
◆ Neurological - low GCS, pain.
◆ Gastrointestinal - nausea and vomiting.

Which patients might require higher levels of monitoring?

Patients having had more major surgery or with concomitant pre-existing cardiorespiratory disease, and those with epidural anaesthesia require more intensive monitoring, such as continuous invasive arterial pressure monitoring and central venous pressure monitoring.

What are the criteria for safe discharge back to the ward?

◆ A - Airway: maintained.
◆ B - Breathing: good respiratory effort, oxygen saturation over 95%.
◆ C - Circulation: cardiovascular observations stable and within normal limits, urine output adequate.
◆ D - Disability: awake and communicative, pain controlled and the patient comfortable. Nausea and vomiting controlled.
◆ E - Everything else: e.g. surgical drains or any special requirements met.

If these criteria are not met what are the options?

Some criteria for not transferring a patient out of recovery might warrant a return to theatre and the surgical team must be contacted urgently; for example, hypovolaemia may be a manifestation of ongoing bleeding requiring a return to theatre. Likewise, ECG changes suggestive of myocardial infarction may require transfer to the coronary care unit. If the patient is stable, but not safe for transfer to a general ward, they will either need to be kept in recovery or transferred for monitoring to an area where a higher level of care can be provided such as the high dependency unit or intensive care unit (see sections 3.9.5 and 3.9.6).

2. Management of immediate postoperative respiratory distress

How is acute airway obstruction recognised?

◆ **Look** - for chest and abdominal movements, cyanosis, respiratory distress, tracheal tug.
◆ **Listen** - for stridor, gurgling, snoring or crowing, wheeze or absent breath sounds.
◆ **Feel** - for air movement at the nose and mouth and chest expansion.
◆ **Use** - the pulse oximeter (see section 2.6.4).

What are the common causes in the postoperative period and what is the management?

◆ Sedative drugs, swelling, bleeding, secretions, laryngospasm.

Management involves manoeuvres to maintain the airway, e.g. head tilt/ chin lift/jaw thrust, suction, high-flow oxygen with a non-rebreath (reservoir) mask or, if there is no respiratory effort, proceed to ventilate with a bag/valve mask and oxygen, and call for help quickly. Consider the use of oropharyngeal or nasopharyngeal airways.

What are the common causes of hypoxaemia in the immediate postoperative period?

◆ Ventilation/perfusion mismatch, e.g. pulmonary oedema, aspiration, pneumothorax, lung collapse, mucous plugging.
◆ Hypoventilation may be due to sedative drugs or residual nerve block.

The management is as above: oxygen by mask, preferably 15 litres per minute with a non-rebreathing mask (reservoir bag). This can deliver up to 85% oxygen; a standard mask can deliver up to 50% oxygen. A venturi mask has a colour coding system which gives an approximation of oxygen concentration delivered (24-60%).

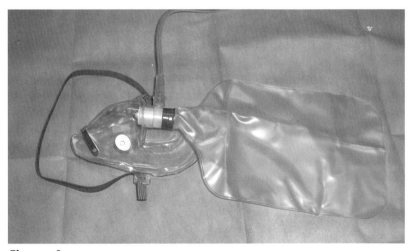

Figure 1. Venturi oxygen mask and reservoir bag.

Why is there confusion about the dangers of too much oxygen?

A MINORITY of patients with chronic obstructive pulmonary disease (COPD) become chronic CO_2 retainers and as such their respiratory centre is driven not by pCO_2 levels, as in the normal healthy population (and the MAJORITY of patients with COPD), but by mild hypoxia. So, if their pO_2 goes up, their respiratory drive falls, their respiratory rate falls and they become hypercapnoeic. These patients may be identified by pre-operative blood gas analysis (raised pCO_2, with compensatory raised bicarbonate).

However, severe hypoxia can be fatal. It is essential to treat severe hypoxaemia immediately with supplemental, high flow oxygen and call for anaesthetic help. If, in the unlikely event that patients are CO_2 retainers, their respiratory rate may fall, their pCO_2 will rise and they may need some ventilatory assistance, but at least they will still be alive when the anaesthetist arrives.

Remember - hypoxia kills before hypercapnia.

3. Management of immediate postoperative hypotension

What are the most significant causes of hypotension in a postoperative setting?

- Hypovolaemia - loss of blood or other fluid with inadequate replacement.
- Compromised cardiac function - arrhythmias or myocardial ischaemia.
- Vasodilatation - drugs, e.g. opiates, sympathetic nervous system blockade, spinal or epidural anaesthesia.

3.9.3

Is hypotension an early or late sign in hypovolaemia?

Hypotension should be considered a late sign in hypovolaemia; a fit healthy person has to lose about 30% of their circulating volume (about 1500ml) before their blood pressure falls, which is class III shock (see below).

What are the early signs of hypovolaemia?

Hypovolaemia causes shock. In early shock or class I shock, the only detectable change is slight anxiety. For class II shock the pulse goes up above 100 beats per minute, the respiratory rate may increase to 20-30 breaths per minute, the diastolic pressure may rise and narrow the pulse pressure, and the patient becomes more anxious. Shock should be recognised and treated at this stage or earlier. Class III shock should be considered a peri-arrest situation and managed aggressively (see section 3.11.14).

What is the management of postoperative hypovolaemia?

Firstly, the diagnosis of postoperative hypovolaemia needs to be confirmed and other causes of postoperative hypotension excluded.

Mild postoperative hypovolaemia can be treated by 'fluid challenge', a bolus of 500ml of fluid (usually normal saline), given intravenously. The pulse/blood pressure/urine output is rechecked after 15 minutes for signs of resolution. If the patient continues to show evidence of hypovolaemia the fluid challenge is repeated, but consideration should be given again to other causes of shock. A central line for measurement of central venous pressure is useful at this stage to guide fluid administration.

Drains, dressings and the operation site are checked for signs of bleeding; beware intra-abdominal bleeding - the abdomen can easily hide 1500ml of blood with no obvious external signs. Blood is sent for haemoglobin concentration and urea and electrolyte estimation.

If the patient remains hypovolaemic, further fluid is administered (blood, crystalloid or colloid) as appropriate, according to the type of fluid loss. This is titrated against pulse, blood pressure, urine output and central pressure.

4. Other recovery room problems

What are the causes of postoperative hypoventilation?

- Sedative drugs - residual anaesthetic effect or as a side effect of analgesics, e.g. opiates.
- Pain - abdominal or thoracic incisions may cause severe pain with breathing, and prevent coughing.
- Residual neuromuscular blockade.
- Reduced respiratory drive, e.g. after forced hyperventilation which reduces the pCO_2.

Management involves supplemental oxygen and treatment of the reversible causes, e.g. naloxone for excess opiates, and consider ventilation if necessary.

What are the possible causes of postoperative hypertension?

Pain, anxiety, urinary retention and a patient who is normally hypertensive. Postoperative hypertension is managed by reassurance, examination of the abdomen for a distended bladder, and ensuring pain is under control. Check the charts for pulse, blood pressure, urine output and pre-operative hypertension.

Why do some patients shiver when they are waking up from an operation?

Shivering can be caused by some volatile anaesthetic agents, but shock and hypothermia are more common causes and need to be excluded. Postoperative hypothermia can put demands on the myocardium and may precipitate myocardial ischaemia.

5. High dependency unit (HDU)

What is a high dependency unit?

A high dependency unit is a ward with a higher level of nursing care and monitoring equipment, suitable for the care of patients with single organ system failure. It is useful for patients requiring closer monitoring than a conventional ward, for example, following major abdominal surgery or myocardial infarction. It is not suitable for patients requiring intensive care unit (ICU) care, haemofiltration or ventilation. The usual patient to nurse ratio is 2:1. The HDU is best placed adjacent to the ICU and staffed by ICU doctors and nurses.

What are the levels of critical care above and below HDU?

- Level 0 - normal ward care.
- Level 1 - enhanced care. Cardiac monitoring, nursing ratio 3:1.
- Level 2 - HDU. Single organ failure (not ventilated), nursing ratio 2:1.
- Level 3 - intensive care. Invasive monitoring, multiple organ failure, ventilation, haemofiltration, nursing ratio 1:1.

A patient's level of care can be escalated or reduced, up and down the scale according to clinical need.

What do you understand by ICU/HDU outreach services?

Outreach services are a ward-based service provided by critical care teams to visit ward patients who are likely to require escalation of care and follow up patients discharged from critical care. They allow easy and early access to skilled care, and are particularly useful when there is a shortage of level 1-3 care beds. They are involved in the education of staff caring for high risk patients in a normal ward setting.

What is the process of escalation of critical care and who is involved?

Escalation of critical care is the process where a patient is moved up through levels 0-3 according to clinical need. It can be initiated by anyone, but is often initiated by a ward nurse or junior doctor by alerting a more senior clinician, or the outreach team.

Escalation is often initiated in response to early warning systems. These are physiological parameters which may be indicated by a patient's routine observations being recorded outside the normal physiological range on the patient's charts (usually hung by or on the patient's bed). They include pulse rate, blood pressure, respiratory rate, temperature, urine output, Glasgow Coma Score, or anything else that makes the ward staff suspicious, e.g. stridor, agitation.

6. Intensive care (ICU or ITU)

When might a postoperative patient need to go to an intensive care unit?

Postoperative ICU admission can be arranged electively (or prophylactically) following major elective surgery, e.g. abdominal aortic aneurysm repair or oesophagectomy, or as an emergency following unexpected medical or surgical complications during surgery. ICU admission for specialised, high level monitoring or treatment should only be arranged for patients with potentially reversible conditions and not for futile situations, such as for patients with advanced malignancy with a very poor prognosis.

Intensive care is requested when mechanical or pharmacological support of organs is required, e.g. ventilation, dialysis, or when more than one organ system has failed. The ICU should be situated on the same floor as, and near to the Accident and Emergency department, theatres and radiology.

3.9.6

When can a postoperative patient be discharged from ICU?

ICU discharge can occur to HDU or to a general ward. Discharge to HDU occurs earlier than to a general ward. Patients need to be discharged to care appropriate for the level of monitoring required in the subsequent postoperative course, e.g. single organ system failure on HDU. Some patients may also be discharged from ICU for terminal care (see section 3.12.6).

The timing of discharge from ICU needs to be decided by senior ICU staff and the surgical consultant responsible for the patient's care.

What ICU scoring systems do you know?

Scoring systems allow comparison between units and hospitals, and evaluation of new treatments, allowing for differences in severity of illness between patients, and prediction of prognosis. The most widely used scoring system is the APACHE system (Acute Physiology And Chronic Health Evaluation). Three versions of this are available (APACHE I, II and III). It has three point scoring components: acute physiology (based on Glasgow Coma Score, blood tests and routine observations), age and chronic disease state.

Other scoring systems include:

◆ SMR - standardised mortality ratio.
◆ SAPS - simplified acute physiology score.
◆ ISS - injury severity score.
◆ RTS - revised trauma score.
◆ TRISS - ratio of RTS and ISS.

Beware - scoring systems are only algorithms and should not be used to influence clinical decision making.

7. Postoperative ventilation

What is ventilation?

Ventilation is the process whereby O_2 is transported to, and CO_2 from, the lungs. In normal life we do this by breathing. Artificial ventilation implies this is done by mechanical means. There are many types of ventilation:

◆ Simple, non-mechanical ventilation, using mouth to mouth, mouth to mask or a bag-valve-mask with or without supplemental oxygen to ventilate a patient.

◆ Intermittent positive pressure ventilation (IPPV). This is the usual mode of ventilation used in theatre and ICU.

◆ Various types of 'controlled' ventilation including pressure-control ventilation (PCV), volume-controlled, intermittent mandatory volume ventilation (IMV), high-frequency ventilation (HFV), high-frequency oscillation (HFO) and high-frequency jet ventilation (HFJV) are sometimes used.

◆ Non-invasive ventilation. This includes constant positive airway pressure (CPAP) ventilation and bi-level positive airways pressure (BiPAP) ventilation. CPAP is when the patient can breathe during expiration but is assisted during inspiration. BiPAP is a two-level CPAP when the patient can breathe, but is assisted during inspiration and expiration. These are non-invasive because the patient does not have an endotracheal tube or laryngeal mask airway; instead there is a tight fitting mask over the mouth and nose.

What is positive end expiratory pressure (PEEP)?

PEEP is a supplement to many modes of ventilation and involves keeping the airway pressure at the end of expiration above ambient pressure. It can help treat atelectasis and maintain alveolar patency but high levels of PEEP may impede venous return to the heart (preload) and impair cardiac output. PEEP is measured in centimetres of water.

Which patients may require prolonged postoperative ventilation?

◆ When the patient is being kept ventilated for a specific reason not related to any problem with their lungs or chest wall or respiratory centre, e.g. after head injury, after head and neck microvascular surgery or following surgery for ruptured aortic aneurysm, to achieve tight control of physiological parameters.

◆ When the patient cannot ventilate themselves but there is no lung disease or chest wall problem, e.g. following neurosurgery.

◆ When the patient can ventilate but due to lung or chest wall disease cannot maintain adequate ventilation, for example, in a patient with pulmonary oedema, aspiration pneumonia or with pre-existing COPD, they may need a prolonged period of postoperative ventilation before they can be weaned off the ventilator.

What is ventilatory weaning?

Weaning is the discontinuation or withdrawal process from mechanical ventilation. It involves balancing the resolution of the conditions which necessitated ventilation with the process of withdrawal of ventilatory support. Delays in weaning can lead to ventilatory complications such as pneumonia, but too rapid withdrawal can lead to hypoxia and potentially dangerous urgent re-intubation. It is a process which depends on accurate assessment of the patient's condition, blood gases, chest radiograph and clinical experience. For successful weaning a patient should be pain-free, cardiovascularly stable, with normal oxygen concentrations and a normal respiratory rate.

Chapter 10

Postoperative ward care

1. Ward rounds

Why do surgeons do postoperative ward rounds?

The care of a patient after surgery is just as important as the operation itself. The postoperative ward round is an important way of ensuring that the postoperative care is correct. This can be best achieved by visiting the patient and the staff who will be responsible for the patient postoperatively and talking to them, answering questions and making sure they understand what is required - have they looked at the operation notes and postop care instruction; is it all clear? The surgeon should also ensure that nothing has changed adversely since leaving theatre, e.g. drains may be clamped or placed at the wrong height, or the patient may not be positioned correctly. A postoperative visit can also be reassuring for the patient and relatives.

Postoperative ward rounds should be performed at the end of the operating list to ensure that the patient is recovering well before the surgical team leave the site, and on the following day and subsequent days, to ensure satisfactory progress. The postoperative ward rounds ensure that procedures, e.g. removal of drains, are performed correctly and also help the discharge team to facilitate discharge planning.

3.10.1

If the operating surgeon is unavailable where can essential information be obtained?

Clear legible operation notes including postoperative instructions are essential and should always be read by the postoperative care team even if the surgeon has done a ward round. If there are other uncertainties the on-call surgical team should be called.

Who should be present on postoperative ward rounds?

The round should consist of one or several of the operating team, depending on their seniority, and someone responsible for the postoperative nursing care of the patient. In an ideal world the on-call junior doctor should also be present.

2. Principles of postoperative analgesia

Why is postoperative pain relief important?

Postoperative pain is the unpleasant sensory and emotional experience due to actual or potential tissue damage following a surgical procedure. It is usually due to the wound, but can be related to patient positioning, lines and catheters or psychological factors. Normally, pain sensation is a protective mechanism, but postoperative pain, although expected, is often detrimental to recovery and may cause further complications. It should be relieved.

The hazards of untreated postoperative pain include:

- General - tachycardia, hypertension, anxiety, fear, insomnia.
- Respiratory - shallow breathing predisposing to atelectasis and chest infection.
- Abdominal - including urinary retention, constipation, reduced appetite.
- Immobility - leading to prolonged hospital stay, DVT risk and chest infection.

What are the principles of management of postoperative pain?

Postoperative analgesia may not completely abolish pain, but aims to promote patient comfort, rapid recovery and rehabilitation. Prevention of potential postoperative pain is better than waiting until the pain is established.

The analgesic ladder is an escalation of pain relief and can be used to assess postoperative pain levels. Patients are started on simple analgesia, and more powerful agents are introduced until pain is under control. This is not ideal for postoperative pain, as it is better to treat potential rather than established pain.

Combination therapy using multiple drugs or modalities is commonly used to treat postoperative pain. Its benefit is that it provides maximum efficacy with minimum toxicity This is in part because different analgesic agents work in different ways and partly due to drug synergism.

The Acute Pain Service (APS) is a multi-disciplinary ward round-based team including doctors, nurses, pharmacists and physiotherapists that are responsible for the day-to-day management of patients with postoperative pain. They are responsible for assessing pain and initiating treatment regimes, including the protocol-driven ongoing care for epidural and patient-controlled analgesia.

How is postoperative pain assessed?

Postoperative pain experience is very subjective. Assessment can be made from a patient's perception of pain, verbally or usually using visual analogue scales. In patients unable to communicate, pain experience can be extrapolated from observation of the patient's manner, or by indirect assessment, e.g. fluctuations in blood pressure, vital capacity, etc.

3. Methods of postoperative analgesia

What methods of postoperative pain relief are available?

3.10.3

◆ Simple oral analgesia - e.g. paracetamol and non-steroidal anti-inflammatory drugs (NSAIDs), such as aspirin and ibuprofen.
◆ Local anaesthetic drugs - administered topically, e.g. EMLA™ cream or injected subcutaneously or in nerve blocks (see section 2.6.6).
◆ Parenteral injected analgesia - subcutaneous, intramuscular or intravenous - can be given by bolus injection or continuous infusion.
◆ Opioid analgesia (see section 2.6.1).
◆ Spinal and epidural anaesthesia (see section 2.6.5).
◆ Patient-controlled analgesia (PCA).

What is PCA?

PCA is a commonly used and effective method of postoperative analgesia. It works by a controlled, intravenous bolus of analgesia, usually opiate, being administered via a pump programmed to deliver specific preset volumes in response to a patient-controlled stimulus, usually a button.

The patient is first given a loading dose of opiate analgesia, sufficient to achieve adequate pain relief; the patient merely administers 'top-up' boluses to maintain analgesia, in response to pain, or anticipation of pain. A timer prevents the administration of a subsequent bolus for a preset time (the lock-out interval). A maximum dose limit can also be preset.

What are the advantages and disadvantages of PCA?

PCA is effective and efficient. The administered doses exactly match the patient's requirement, avoiding the need for painful intramuscular injections and saving nurse time.

It is, however, unsuitable for drowsy or disorientated patients, or those unable to self-administer the dose. Careful monitoring is required. The equipment is expensive and technical errors can be fatal.

4. Mechanisms of postoperative analgesia

How does paracetamol work and what are the side effects?

Paracetamol is a mild oral or intravenous analgesic and antipyretic. It has no significant anti-inflammatory activity. The exact mechanism of action is uncertain.

Side effects are rare and include rashes, blood dyscrasias and liver damage. Overdose can cause serious liver damage and can be fatal.

How do NSAIDs work and what are their side effects?

NSAIDs include aspirin, diclofenac and ibuprofen. They are analgesic, anti-inflammatory and antipyretic. They work by blocking the cyclo-oxygenase pathway, preventing prostaglandin synthesis. Prostaglandins are the mediators causing pain receptors to register noxious stimuli.

Side effects include gastric irritation, peptic ulceration, renal failure, bruising and bleeding, and bronchospasm. Also beware drug interactions, especially with warfarin.

How does opioid analgesia work and what are the side effects?

Opioid analgesics include codeine, morphine and its derivatives, and fentanyl. They are analgesics, mood elevators and anxiolytics. They act at opioid receptors in the brain and peripheral nervous system, blocking neural transmission in pain pathways. They are available orally, subcutaneously, intramuscularly and intravenously, or can be used in spinal or epidural blocks, as boluses or by continuous infusion.

Side effects include nausea and vomiting, respiratory depression, constipation, urinary retention and hypotension. Opioid analgesics may also rarely precipitate tolerance and addiction.

5. Fluid and electrolyte balance

Why do postoperative patients develop electrolyte abnormalities?

3.10.5

Pre-operative: patients have usually taken nothing by mouth for a few hours and may be dehydrated.

Peri-operatively: intravenous fluid administration will affect the patient's electrolyte composition. The patient's normal homeostatic mechanisms may be disrupted. The kidneys may function abnormally often due to hypoperfusion which affects sodium, potassium and pH control. The lungs are important for pH control through CO_2 levels and this can be affected by under- or over-ventilation. Metabolism in the tissues can also be abnormal, for example, under-perfused tissues undergo anaerobic metabolism and cause an increase in potassium and a fall in serum pH. Patients in septic shock will have a generalised under-perfusion of their tissues and may become very acidotic.

Peri-operative and postoperative patients may lose a lot of electrolyte-rich fluid which affects electrolyte levels; for example, vomiting may lead to a hyponatraemic alkalosis, fistulae can cause a massive loss of electrolytes especially sodium and potassium, as can diarrhoea.

Why is the serum potassium concentration important?

Potassium is the major cation (positive ion) of the intracellular fluid. It is actively pumped into the cell to create a concentration gradient across the cell membrane. Diffusion of potassium out of the cell down this concentration gradient is responsible for the resting membrane potential of nerves and muscles. Potassium is not greatly affected by water loss or retention but factors which affect the potassium concentration gradient, by moving potassium into or out of the cell have a significant effect on the resting membrane potential. Cellular potassium uptake is stimulated by insulin and there is a reciprocal relationship between potassium and hydrogen ions (acid). Therefore, when the acidity goes up (pH falls), the potassium ions are displaced from the cell to maintain electroneutrality and the patient becomes hyperkalaemic.

Because of the relationship between the potassium concentration gradient and resting membrane potential of excitable cells, the effects of abnormal potassium levels are serious, even with seemingly small changes. Hence, the normal serum range is narrow. Hyperkalaemia and hypokalaemia cause muscle weakness and cardiac arrhythmias and may cause cardiac arrest.

How do you calculate the fluid requirements in a postoperative patient?

♦ History - pre-existing medical conditions, especially renal disease and heart failure. What surgery has been performed, how long did it take, and what fluids were given? etc.

♦ Examination - pulse, blood pressure, urine output, respiratory rate, jugular venous pressure or central venous pressure, tissue turgor and oedema. Check drips and lines are functioning, and that the drains are not blocked or draining excessive amounts.

♦ Investigations - biochemical tests are no substitute for history and examination. Electrolyte, urea and creatinine concentrations should be performed.

♦ Estimation - fluid replacement can be given enterally when feasible, but many postoperative patients are unable to take adequate oral fluids, so it is necessary to prescribe intravenous fluids. The fundamental principles are to make up for lost fluid and electrolytes, and provide maintenance fluid. For maintenance, an adult requires approximately 2.5 litres of water, plus 2mmol/kg sodium and 1mmol/kg potassium. In your calculation you must include not just your estimated deficit and maintenance requirements, but also the insensible losses.

What are insensible losses and how are they estimated?

Insensible losses are those which cannot normally be measured and include normal faeces (100-200ml), respiratory losses (500-700ml) and sweat (200-400ml) per day. Insensible loss is affected by pyrexia, tachypnoea, ambient temperature, mechanical ventilation or even just giving un-humidified oxygen via a face mask. The reality is you are unlikely to be accurate in your estimation of insensible losses but you must bear it in mind, make an estimation, try a regimen and reassess the patient regularly and their response will tell you if you are getting it right.

6. Management of postoperative oliguria

What is oliguria?

3.10.6

Oliguria is urine output of less than 400ml in 24 hours, or less then 0.5ml/kg/hour in an adult.

In practice urine output of less than 30ml/hour for three consecutive hours is treated as oliguria. Anuria is the total absence of urine output.

What are the causes of postoperative oliguria?

◆ Pre-renal causes. Hypovolaemia is the commonest cause of postoperative oliguria. This can be due to blood loss, plasma loss (burns) or water loss (dehydration, diarrhoea, vomiting). Other possible pre-renal causes include septic shock, anaphylactic shock, low output cardiac failure, epidural analgesia, renal artery stenosis and raised intra-abdominal pressure (abdominal compartment syndrome).

◆ Renal causes. These include acute tubular necrosis following prolonged hypotension (e.g. ruptured abdominal aortic aneurysm repair), and nephrotoxic drugs (e.g. gentamicin). Pre-existing causes of postoperative renal failure manifest as oliguria should also be considered (e.g. glomerulonephritis, hypertension, vasculitis).

◆ Post-renal causes. The commonest cause is a blocked catheter (this usually causes anuria rather than oliguria). Other possible causes include ureteric stones or fibrosis, and bladder outflow obstruction caused by an enlarged prostate (of any cause), stones or a stricture.

What is the management of postoperative oliguria?

Firstly a catheter is passed, if not already present, to exclude retention, and for accurate urine output measurement. If a catheter is present it should be flushed to exclude blockage. Other non-hypovolaemic causes of oliguria need to be excluded or treated.

Hypovolaemia and hypotension are then corrected, by boluses of intravenous fluid; a central venous pressure catheter can be used to monitor the responses of the fluid challenge (see sections 3.9.3 and 3.11.14). When optimal filling is achieved, as measured by central venous pressure or pulmonary artery pressure, inotropes, or vasopressor agents can be administered to promote adequate renal perfusion, or diuretics used to promote diuresis. A urine output greater than 30ml/hour should be the aim.

Other contributing factors should also be identified and prevented, e.g. NSAIDs, ACE inhibitors, gentamicin.

If these measures fail the patient should be transferred to HDU/ICU for consideration of haemofiltration or dialysis.

7. Wound healing (pathology)

What are the phases of wound healing?

◆ Stage 1 - inflammation - acute inflammatory response with vasoconstriction, then vasodilatation and coagulation. Immune cells remove dead tissue and bacteria (day 0-7).
◆ Stage 2 - proliferation - vascular proliferation, collagen synthesis and epithelialisation - either from the wound edges or from the epithelial

lining of hair follicles and sweat glands. Myofibroblasts cause wound contraction (day 1 to week 3).

◆ Stage 3 - remodelling and scar maturation - collagen remodelling and maturation (week 3 to 1 year).

What is granulation tissue?

It is a tissue involved in the process of tissue repair. It is composed of loops of capillaries supported by myofibroblasts. Its name originates from the granular appearance of the tissue due to the capillary loops.

What is scar tissue?

When specialised tissue is destroyed and cannot be replaced, a process of repair occurs and scar tissue is the resultant tissue. Its exact composition depends upon the degree of scar maturation. A young scar is composed of granulation tissue. A mature scar is predominantly fibrous tissue. Scars do not contain melanin. In the central nervous system scars are formed of glial tissue.

What is the difference between hypertrophic and keloid scars?

Hypertrophic scars are abnormally large scars due to excessive fibroblast proliferation but are confined to the wound margins. Keloids are proliferative scars infiltrating beyond wound margins. Hypertrophic scars usually diminish with time. Keloid scars are commoner in Afro-Caribbeans, and on the chest wall. They recur following excision. They can be improved after steroid infiltration into the scar tissue.

8. Factors affecting wound healing

What factors impair wound healing?

Local factors:

- Inadequate blood supply.
- Excessive skin tension.
- Poor wound apposition.
- Wound breakdown.
- Foreign body.
- Infection.
- Excessive wound mobility, such as over a joint or a moving tendon.
- Radiotherapy.

Systemic factors:

- Malnutrition.
- Smoking.
- Diabetes.
- Obesity.
- Chemotherapy.
- Immunosuppression.
- Immunocompromise.
- Steroids.
- Deficiency of vitamins and trace elements.
- Genetic disorders, e.g. leucocyte adhesion deficiency.

What are the risk factors for unsightly scarring?

All of the above plus a history of keloid formation and wounds running across relaxed skin lines or across important anatomical lines, such as the eyelids or vermilion border of the lip.

3.10.8

9. Postoperative nutrition

3.10.9

Why are some patients kept 'nil by mouth' following surgical procedures?

In the immediate postoperative period, especially after general anaesthesia, many patients feel drowsy or nauseated. Although postoperative oral fluids and diet may not be contraindicated, patients may feel more comfortable if they are not expected to eat or drink during this period.

Patients having had gastrointestinal surgery may have a postoperative ileus, so diet and fluids may be restricted during this time to prevent nausea and vomiting. However, there is considerable evidence that early enteral feeding speeds recovery. Patients who have had head and neck surgery, oesophageal or gastric surgery may not be able to eat in the postoperative period.

Which patients require postoperative nutritional support?

Postoperative nutritional support is required by patients who cannot eat, e.g. following major head and neck, oesophageal or gastric surgery; or in patients with hypermetabolic states, e.g. following other complex surgery, burns, major trauma or sepsis. Support is also required for patients unable to tolerate enteral feeding, e.g. inflammatory bowel diseases, prolonged ileus, gastrointestinal fistulae, pancreatitis and malabsorption states. It may be beneficial to commence postoperative nutrition in the immediate postoperative period. This requires pre-operative planning.

What routes of postoperative nutrition are available?

Conventional oral feeding is the best form of nutrition for those in whom it is possible, with dietary supplements if appropriate.

Enteral nutrition is indicated in patients who are unable to feed conventionally, but have a functioning gastrointestinal (GI) tract. For short-term feeding (4-6 weeks), a fine bore nasogastric or nasojejunal tube feed is used. For longer-term nutrition, a percutaneous endoscopic gastrostomy (PEG), surgical feeding gastrostomy or surgical feeding jejunostomy is required.

Complications of enteral tube feeding include tube malposition, blockage or displacement, aspiration, peri-stomal leakage leading to peritonitis or skin irritation, diarrhoea, nausea and vomiting, bloating, and vitamin, mineral or trace element deficiencies.

When the GI tract is non-functional, total parenteral nutrition (TPN) is the feeding method of choice. This is intravenous feeding via a central or peripheral vein. Monitoring of TPN is required (daily blood count, U+Es, glucose, weekly liver function tests, albumin, trace elements and vitamins). Complications include fluid overload, deficiency states and complications of central lines (see section 2.7.2). Most hospitals have a dietition department and a TPN team who will oversee postoperative nutrition.

10. Stomas

What types of stoma do you know?

A stoma is a surgically created connection between a visceral lumen and the skin.

- Colostomy - this stoma is between the colon and the abdominal wall skin. It can be an end colostomy or loop colostomy. An end colostomy is usually performed following abdominoperineal resection of the rectum for rectal or anal cancer, or following Hartmann's procedure for colonic obstruction or perforation. They usually lie in the left iliac fossa. A loop (or side) colostomy is usually performed to defunction (or rest) the distal colon following colonic anastomosis. It is usually found in the right upper quadrant.
- Ileostomy - is a stoma between the small bowel and the abdominal wall skin. An end ileostomy is usually in the right iliac fossa, and has a spout to protect the skin from small bowel content. It is performed following total colectomy for inflammatory bowel diseases or tumours.

3.10.10

A loop (side) ileostomy is also usually in the right iliac fossa and has a similar function to loop colostomy.

◆ Urostomy - is a stoma between the ureter(s) and the abdominal wall, usually joined via an isolated section of small bowel. It is performed following cystectomy to allow external urine drainage.

◆ Nephrostomy - is an artificial connection between the pelvis of the kidney and the skin, via a plastic tube. It is used to drain the kidney with ureteric obstruction that cannot be relieved by other less invasive techniques.

◆ Tracheostomy - (see section 3.10.11).

◆ Gastostomy - is a stoma between stomach lumen and abdominal wall skin used for feeding or gastric decompression (see section 3.10.9)

◆ Jejunostomy - is a stoma between jejunal lumen and abdominal wall skin used for feeding (see section 3.10.9).

◆ Laparostomy - is the name given to a laparotomy wound left open with the viscera covered in a plastic sheet or moist gauze, to treat infection or abdominal compartment syndrome (see section 3.11.17)

What is the role of a stoma nurse?

A stoma nurse is especially trained to manage colostomy, ileostomy and urostomy and teach patients how to do so. These stoma have bags for collection of visceral content: stool, small bowel content or urine, respectively. They need to be emptied regularly and the skin around the stoma cared for to prevent damage. Stoma nurses teach the patients how to apply and empty the bags.

11. Tracheostomy

What is the difference between a tracheostomy and a tracheotomy?

The terms are commonly used interchangeably, although -otomy means a surgical incision into something and -ostomy means a surgically created opening between two organs or an organ and skin. Therefore, some surgeons refer to tracheotomy as a temporary procedure and a tracheostomy as a longer-term procedure.

What are the purposes of each procedure?

Temporary tracheotomies are elective or urgent, either because a surgical procedure requires a bypass of the upper airway, or because a maxillofacial injury or disease process requires it. A permanent tracheostomy is usually performed following a major resection of the larynx or occasionally due to congenital abnormalities and rarely as a palliative procedure.

Percutaneous tracheotomy is a procedure usually performed on an ICU by an anaesthetist as an aid to weaning a ventilated patient. It is performed by introducing a percutaneous dilator over a guidewire to allow introduction of a tracheostomy tube.

There is some disagreement over the concept of 'emergency tracheotomies' but it is important to remember that a tracheotomy is not an acceptable operation for a patient in respiratory arrest; that requires a cricothyroidotomy: a temporary emergency airway established by inserting a tube through the cricothyroid membrane. However, there is still some debate about whether a tracheotomy is an acceptable intervention for a patient with severe upper airways obstruction; it depends on the circumstances and the surgeon. There is no doubt that in almost all situations a cricothyroidotomy is the quickest, safest and easiest way to gain access to the airway in an emergency.

What are the major intra-operative complications of these procedures?

Bleeding, tracheal damage, pneumothorax, haemothorax, malpositioning of the tracheal airway, and loss of airway resulting in asphyxia and death. Long-term complications include tracheal stenosis which may necessitate further surgery or a long-term tracheostomy.

12. Chest drains

What are the indications for insertion of a chest drain?

A chest drain is a tube for removal of gas or liquid (effusion, blood, pus) from the pleural cavity, allowing re-expansion of the underlying lung. It has a collection bottle which must be kept below chest level, and is connected via a one-way valve, such as an underwater-seal drainage unit to prevent negative intrathoracic pressure sucking the contents back into the chest.

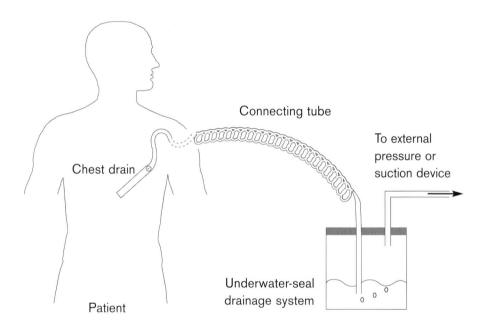

Figure 1. **Chest drain.**

Emergency indications include: tension pneumothorax (after needle thoracocentesis); pneumothorax in a ventilated patient; traumatic large haemothorax or pneumothorax; and empyema.

Less urgent indications include persistent pneumothorax despite needle aspiration, large spontaneous pneumothorax, large pleural effusions and post-thoracic surgery, e.g. oesophagectomy, cardiac surgery.

How is a chest drain inserted?

This is performed under local anaesthesia using aseptic technique. A short incision is made over the 4th or 5th intercostal space in the mid-axillary line. Blunt dissection is performed to the pleural cavity, at the upper border of the rib to avoid damage to the intercostal vessels and nerves, and a finger is inserted to ensure entry to the pleural cavity. The drain is inserted without the sharp obturator and secured in position with a stitch. The wound is dressed with an occlusive dressing and the drainage tube connected to the underwater-seal drainage unit.

What are the complications of chest drains?

"There is no organ in the thoracic or abdominal cavity that has not been pierced by a chest drain."

Complications of insertion:

♦ Haemothorax.
♦ Lung laceration.
♦ Cardiac injury.
♦ Diaphragmatic injury causing abdominal cavity penetration.
♦ Subcutaneous placement.

Later complications:

♦ Tube displacement or blockage.
♦ Retained haemothorax.
♦ Wound infection.
♦ Empyema.
♦ Persistant pneumothorax after removal.

Chapter 11

Postoperative complications

1. Classification of postoperative complications

How do you classify postoperative complications?

◆ Immediate - complications occurring at or immediately after surgery in the recovery room, e.g. postoperative airway obstruction (see section 3.9.2).
◆ Early - complications occurring within 48 hours of surgery, e.g. reactive haemorrhage (see section 3.11.13).
◆ Late - complications occurring 48 hours or more after surgery, e.g. pressure ulceration (see section 3.12.3).

Complications can be specific to the operation, e.g. recurrent laryngeal nerve injury following thyroidectomy, or general, e.g. bleeding, wound infection.

What are the risk factors for postoperative complications?

◆ Emergency surgery.
◆ Surgery performed out of normal working hours.
◆ Old age.
◆ Malnutrition.

3.11.1

- ◆ Smoking.
- ◆ Diabetes.
- ◆ Obesity.
- ◆ Ischaemic heart disease.
- ◆ Chemotherapy.
- ◆ Immunosuppression.
- ◆ Steroids.

What steps can be taken to reduce the incidence and consequences of postoperative complications?

Prophylaxis: e.g. DVT prophylaxis, antibiotic prophylaxis (see section 1.3.6). A high index of suspicion is required to anticipate potential postoperative problems to allow earlier intervention, e.g. empirical antibiotic treatment for a wound with early and subtle signs of infection can reduce the extent of tissue damage and reduce subsequent complications, such as wound breakdown and sepsis.

2. Postoperative pyrexia

What is normal core temperature?

3.11.2

Normal body temperature varies slightly between individuals but is generally around 37°C. Core temperature is best measured by an ear probe; oral and rectal temperatures are usually slightly cooler. Postoperative pyrexia is a manifestation of the body's increased metabolic rate in response to inflammation, trauma or infection.

What are the common causes of postoperative pyrexia?

Low grade postoperative pyrexia can be part of the normal response to trauma. Persistent, relapsing, or high grade pyrexia can be due to:

- ◆ Wound infection.
- ◆ Chest infection.
- ◆ Urinary tract infection.

- Abscess formation - usually a high grade swinging pyrexia.
- DVT or PE.
- Infected pressure area sores.
- Infected lines, drips or tubes.
- Malignancy.
- Other - bacterial endocarditis, myocardial infarction (MI).

How would you investigate postoperative pyrexia?

- Check the wound.
- Chest X-ray.
- Sputum culture.
- Blood culture.
- Check the calves, examine for stigmata of DVT/PE.
- Urine analysis and culture.
- Check pressure areas.
- Check all lines, drips and tubes for signs of infection.

If the cause is not apparent blood is sent for culture and further investigation may be required, e.g. ultrasound or CT scan to exclude intra-abdominal collection.

3. Postoperative wound infection

What are the symptoms and signs of wound infection?

Wound infection manifests itself with the cardinal signs of acute inflammation:

- Rubor - redness.
- Calor - warmth.
- Dolor - pain.
- Tumor - swelling.
- Loss of function.

The wound edges may begin to come apart and there may be a discharge from the wound (clear, bloody or purulent).

3.11.3

How is an infected wound managed?

Mild wound infections may resolve spontaneously. More serious wound infections, with signs of inflammation, may require antibiotics. Initially, broad-spectrum antibiotics are administered; these can be changed later to targeted antibiotics based on sensitivities to cultured organisms.

In serious wound infections, or when there is a suspicion of a collection of pus, the wound needs to be laid open or a few sutures need to be removed. The defect can then be allowed to heal by secondary intention (see section 2.8.1), or re-sutured when clean at a later date.

Chronic wound infections may require debridement. This can be done surgically with a scalpel, chemically with topical de-sloughing agents, or biologically with maggots (larvae therapy).

What sorts of wounds are most likely to get infected?

Contaminated and dirty wounds (see section 1.3.6), traumatic wounds, irregular and complex wounds.

What are the risk factors for wound infection?

Local factors:

◆ Inadequate blood supply.
◆ Excessive skin tension.
◆ Foreign body.
◆ Poor hygiene.

Systemic factors (see section 1.2):

◆ Malnutrition.
◆ Diabetes.
◆ Obesity.
◆ Malignancy.

4. Wound dehiscence

What is wound dehiscence?

Wound dehiscence is unplanned spontaneous re-opening of a wound following surgical closure. Partial dehiscence is the re-opening of the skin and superficial tissues; full dehiscence is total wound re-opening, so the floor of the wound or contents of the underlying cavity are exposed, e.g. burst abdomen.

What factors predispose to wound dehiscence?

◆ Wound infection - superficial wound infection causes local ischaemia, preventing normal wound healing and allowing wound dehiscence. Deeper wound infections or abscess formation may discharge through the wound causing dehiscence. Dirty wounds or wounds with implanted foreign bodies are at higher risk of dehiscence.

◆ Poor surgical technique - poor surgical wound closure technique can lead to dehiscence (see section 2.8.4); for example, sutures placed too far apart or too close to the wound edge may 'cut out'. Wounds closed under too much tension or with poor wound edge apposition will also tend to re-open.

◆ Poor blood supply - healing wounds require a good blood supply to facilitate healing; hence, wounds in ischaemic feet may fail to heal. Inferior-based flaps on extremities also may have poor blood supply.

◆ Premature suture removal - skin sutures in adults should be left in for five days (face, arms), one week (chest, abdomen), ten to fourteen days (back, legs). Sutures can be removed earlier in children and should be left longer in areas of poor healing, e.g. ischaemic extremities.

◆ General factors include malnutrition, steroids, obesity, malignancy, jaundice, elderly patients, anaemia, diabetes, immunosuppression.

3.11.4

How is wound dehiscence managed?

◆ Deep layers - re-suture with good surgical technique.
◆ Superficial layers - re-suture if clean or leave to heal by secondary intention (see section 2.8.1).

What is the difference between a sinus and a fistula?

A fistula is an abnormal connection between two epitheliased surfaces, e.g. fistula-in-ano; an abnormal connection between perineal skin and anal mucosa.

A sinus is a blind-ending tract leading from an epitheliased surface, e.g. pilonidal sinus, a tract usually containing hair, opening in the natal cleft.

5. Postoperative deep vein thrombosis (DVT)

Why do patients get postoperative DVT?

DVT is thrombus in the deep veins of the legs. It is a common postoperative complication. Thrombosis risks relate to Virchow's triad:

◆ Stasis - postoperative immobility allows venous pooling leading to stasis and DVT.
◆ Vessel wall - extrinsic compression of deep veins, e.g. following orthopaedic or abdominal surgery.
◆ Blood constituents - blood may be hypercoagulable in postoperative patients, with dehydration or malignancy.

What are the risk factors for DVT?

Immobility, trauma, age, obesity, malignancy, previous DVT, pregnancy, contraceptive pill, smoking, thrombophilia, dehydration (see section 1.3.5).

What are the symptoms and signs?

Many postoperative DVTs are asymptomatic. DVT can present with a painful, red, swollen, tender, slightly warm calf or leg and low grade systemic pyrexia. DVT can present as pulmonary embolism (see section 3.11.6).

How is the diagnosis made?

This is initially a clinical diagnosis, based on symptoms and signs, and a high index of suspicion. The diagnosis can usually be confirmed on colour duplex Doppler ultrasonography. Occasionally, a venogram is required in difficult cases.

What are the complications of DVT?

◆ Pulmonary embolism - an immediate or early serious complication.
◆ Post-phlebitic leg - presents many months or years later with a swollen, painful leg, skin changes of chronic venous disease or ulceration.

DVT prophylaxis (see section 1.3.5).

6. Pulmonary embolism (PE)

Why do surgeons need to know about pulmonary emboli?

Pulmonary embolus is an important postoperative complication following deep venous thrombosis. Part or all of the thrombus in the leg veins is propelled through the venous system, inferior vena cava and right side of the heart, and impacts in the pulmonary arteries causing partial or total occlusion.

3.11.6

What are the symptoms and signs of pulmonary emboli?

Small pulmonary emboli may be asymptomatic. Some small or moderate PE may present with pleuritic chest pain, shortness of breath, haemoptysis and symptoms of hypoxia. Signs include cyanosis, tachycardia, pleural rub and low grade pyrexia. Some PE present more insidiously with signs of right heart strain. Large PE may present with sudden onset severe shortness of breath, collapse and sudden death.

How is the diagnosis made?

A high index of suspicion is required in postoperative patients with respiratory problems. Investigation includes blood gas analysis confirming hypoxia, an ECG (unreliable) which may show evidence of right heart strain with classic S1 Q3 T3 changes and a ventilation/perfusion (VQ) scan. The most reliable method of diagnosis is CT pulmonary angiography.

What are the treatment options?

Immediate management involves oxygen by mask, intravenous fluids and anticoagulation, initially with intravenous or subcutaneous heparin. After diagnostic confirmation full anticoagulation with warfarin is required. Indications for a vena caval filter include ongoing pulmonary emboli despite adequate anticoagulation and loose or free-floating thrombus in the leg or pelvic veins as diagnosed on Doppler ultrasound. Other treatments include thrombolysis.

7. Postoperative myocardial infarction (MI)

What are the symptoms and signs of a postoperative MI?

Postoperative MI can present in unusual ways and a high index of suspicion is required. It may not present with typical retrosternal chest pain radiating to the arm or neck. Many present without any pain at all, with recent onset heart failure (raised JVP, pulmonary oedema, hypotension) or

3.11.7

arrhythmias, especially tachycardia or bradycardia. Nausea, vomiting, or tachypnoea may be present.

The signs may include pallor, cold and clammy skin, a gallop rhythm, lung crepitations and occasionally pyrexia. Patients may even tell you that they 'just feel awful'.

What is the most usual time for a postoperative MI?

About two thirds occur around day two to five but they can occur at any time; be suspicious especially in high risk patients.

What is the immediate management of a suspected MI?

ABC of course! Perform an ECG and administer supplemental oxygen. Monitor blood pressure, pulse and respiratory rate, obtain venous access and arrange appropriate blood tests including T troponin (mnemonic: ABC what's on the ECG?).

Then, if you still suspect an MI give some sublingual glyceryl tri-nitrate (GTN) and aspirin, and if necessary give some morphine and an antiemetic, and GET HELP (mnemonic: MONA, Morphine, Oxygen, Nitrates, Aspirin).

What is the medium and long-term management?

The patient should see a cardiologist within the first hour whenever possible, and should be considered for anti-thrombotic therapy, coronary artery stenting or even coronary artery bypass grafts, although these options are often limited in the immediate postoperative patient. Additional long-term management includes medical treatments (beta-blockers, ACE inhibitors, aspirin, statins) and behavioral lifestyle modification (counselling, exercise, dietary changes).

What is thought to be the most dangerous interval after having an MI to undergo surgery?

The risk of having another MI after elective surgery is about 35% in the first three months after the original MI, and 15% in the next three to six months. After six months it is about 4%. Therefore, elective surgery should be avoided where possible for at least the first six months. The mortality from re-infarction may be as high as 30-40%.

8. Postoperative stroke

Why do strokes occur after surgery?

Strokes or cerebrovascular accidents (CVA) are due to an interruption to the blood supply to the brain or an intracerebral bleed. Many of the risk factors for CVA can occur around the time of surgery: hypertension as a response to pain; hypotension due to anaesthesia or hypovolaemia; hypercoagulability due to dehydration; and hypocoagulability due to the use of heparin. Also, arrhythmias such as atrial fibrillation are common postoperatively, and can precipitate thromboembolic CVA. Some operations, such as carotid endarterectomy and neck dissections, can dislodge thrombus and cause a thromboembolic CVA. Other surgical procedures, often vascular, where the blood clotting time is iatrogenically prolonged, increase the risk of haemorrhagic CVA.

What are the symptoms and signs?

Strokes present as a rapid onset of focal neurological signs and symptoms or a progressive step-wise deterioration of neurological function. The symptoms and signs may be localising, that is the affected vessel is supplying a particular part of the brain with a specific function, but collateral supply can complicate presentation. The most commonly affected vessel is a branch of the middle cerebral artery which supplies the internal capsule. This causes contralateral hemiplegia, hemisensory loss, facial muscle weakness and hemianopia.

3.11.8

What investigations are helpful?

After a full history and examination with special emphasis on the neurological system and routine pulse and blood pressure, the basic work up should include full blood count, coagulation profile, ECG, blood glucose and lipids. Ultrasound imaging of the heart (ECHO) and the carotid arteries may be useful in selected cases. MRI or CT imaging of the brain is now advised in all cases where there are grounds to suspect a CVA.

What treatments might be indicated?

If the stroke is diagnosed quickly and the scan shows it is a thromboembolic type, then anti-thrombotic therapy may be appropriate, but often this is not an option postoperatively due to the risk of wound bleeding. Haemorrhagic stroke should be treated by correcting any clotting abnormality to prevent further deterioration.

9. Postoperative chest infection

What is pneumonia?

Pneumonia is inflammation of the lung parenchyma. Chest infection is a broader term as it includes inflammation of the bronchi and trachea, caused by infection.

3.11.9

What are the risk factors for aspiration pneumonia?

In surgical patients, aspiration pneumonia as a result of aspirating the gastric contents (Mendelson's syndrome) may occur during general anaesthesia. The risk factors for this are intubation of a patient without normal pre-operative fasting in emergency or trauma situations, or when the patient is at high risk of gastro-oesophageal reflux, such as pregnant and obese patients, and those with hiatus hernia.

Patients are also at risk of developing aspiration pneumonia postoperatively. This may include gastric contents but also saliva or food during eating. This is particularly likely if they have disordered swallowing such as after surgery to the mouth or pharynx or if they have neurological problems such as stroke, are heavily sedated, are comatose or have Alzheimer's disease.

How is hospital-acquired pneumonia (HAP) different from community-acquired pneumonia (CAP)?

CAP occurs more often in the winter and is usually due to pathogens either from the upper airways or from infected individuals. The most common pathogen is *Streptococcus pneumoniae*. Patients with chronic obstructive pulmonary disease are more likely to have *Haemophilus influenzae* pneumonia and those who develop CAP after influenza or steroid therapy are more likely to be infected with *Staphylococcus aureus*. The atypical group is a subset involving intracellular organisms such as *Mycobacterium pneumoniae*.

HAP is a new onset pneumonia starting more that 48 hours after hospital admission. It may be due to aspiration of organisms from the nasopharynx, or due to nosocomial infection from equipment, especially ventilation equipment. It may also be due to infective emboli from distant sites. Hospitalised patients are particularly at risk if they have impaired consciousness, an inability to cough and clear secretions, are immunocompromised or have prolonged ventilation. The pathogens involved are a much wider group than CAP and include gram negative bacilli such as *Enterobacter* and *E. coli* and gram positive organisms such as *Streptococcus pneumoniae*. Postoperative HAP is more likely in those at extremes of age, smokers and the obese.

10. Atelectasis and respiratory failure

What is atelectasis?

Atelectasis is collapse of portions of the lung tissue, due to inadequate ventilation of the alveoli and failure to clear pulmonary secretions. It is

3.11.10

common following surgery, especially with upper abdominal and thoracic incisions. Other risk factors include immobility, poor postoperative analgesia, over-sedation, smoking, malnutrition, age, obesity and pre-existing respiratory disease.

A high index of suspicion is required for this complication, especially in patients with the above risk factors. Ideally, patients should stop smoking pre-operatively for elective surgery, and supplementary oxygen and physiotherapy with adequate analgesia should be administered routinely in the early postoperative period. Early mobilisation and minimal postoperative sedation are also required.

Untreated atelectasis can lead to established chest infection requiring antibiotics and aggressive physiotherapy. Later sequelae may include bronchopneumonia and pleural effusions, and may require ventilatory support.

What is respiratory failure?

Respiratory failure occurs when the pulmonary gas exchange is sufficiently impaired to cause hypoxia with or without hypercapnia. There are two types:

- Type 1 - PaO_2 <8kPa and $PaCO_2$ normal or low. This is due to a diffusion defect, a ventilation-perfusion mismatch or a left to right shunt.
- Type 2 - PaO_2 <8kPa and $PaCO_2$ >7kPa (high). This is due to hypoventilation.

What is the most useful investigation in respiratory failure and why?

Arterial blood gas measurement is essential because it gives definitive measurements of the PaO_2 and $PaCO_2$ and leads most quickly to a diagnosis. Blood gas analysis also gives bicarbonate levels which can show if the patient is a chronic CO_2 retainer (respiratory acidosis) as the bicarbonate level will be high due to compensatory renal alkalosis.

11. Postoperative pneumothorax

What are the causes of postoperative pneumothorax?

Pneumothorax may be an incidental result of thoracic surgery and the treatment of the pneumothorax, the chest drain, is a part of the operation. However, accidental or iatrogenic pneumothorax is more dangerous if it is not diagnosed promptly. It can occur after simple procedures such as subclavian central line placement and may gradually develop over a period of time. It is particularly risky after procedures such as bronchial biopsy or rib harvesting but can also occur after any anaesthetic, due to the effects of positive pressure ventilation.

How is it recognised?

In simple pneumothorax there will be dyspnoea, hyper-resonance, absent breath sounds and less chest wall movement on the affected side. The trachea may be deviated towards the affected side and the chest radiograph will show an area devoid of lung markings. Tension pneumothorax is a clinical diagnosis. The patient will be tachycardic, hypotensive and tachypnoeic, and distressed; the chest will be hyper-resonant and have absent breath sounds and reduced movement over the affected side. There will also be deviation of the trachea away from the affected side and the neck veins will be distended. There is no time for a chest radiograph as it requires immediate decompression to avoid cardiac arrest and death.

How is it treated?

Tension pneumothorax requires immediate needle thoracostomy. A Venflon™ is inserted into the thoracic cavity just above the fourth rib in the mid-clavicular line. This will decompress the pneumothorax until definitive treatment with a chest drain can be achieved. Simple pneumothoraces may be treated with aspiration in some circumstances but postoperatively most require a chest drain (see section 3.10.12).

Why are patients with COPD more at risk?

Rupture of emphysematous bullae is a well known complication of positive pressure ventilation in patients with COPD. In men, heavy smokers are over 100 times more likely to develop a pneumothorax than non-smokers.

12. Postoperative bleeding - primary haemorrhage

What is meant by primary haemorrhage?

Primary haemorrhage is bleeding during an operation. Intra-operative bleeding can come from a number of sources:

◆ Arterial bleeding - pulsatile blood flow, e.g. following inadvertent division or damage to an artery during dissection.
◆ Venous bleeding - caused by damage to large veins, e.g. pre-sacral venous bleeding during pelvic dissection.
◆ Capillary bleeding - occurs from large raw areas, e.g. from the liver bed following cholecystectomy.

How is primary haemorrhage controlled?

All bleeding is best initially controlled by pressure. A swab is placed over the bleeding area and firm pressure applied. This will stop small 'bleeders' over the bleeding area and allow the surgeon time to organise the appropriate instruments/sutures to repair larger vessels.

Arterial bleeding is controlled by diathermy for small arterioles (see section 2.7.8) and ligation for bigger vessels when end organ blood supply is not required. Arterial bleeding, when the patency of the artery is to be maintained, is managed by direct suture repair of the damaged vessel whilst bleeding is controlled by proximal and distal (non-crushing) clamps.

Venous bleeding is notoriously more difficult to control and is especially dangerous as large volumes of blood can be rapidly lost. Venous bleeding is best controlled with pressure. Sometimes it is possible to directly re-suture or under-run bleeding veins, but care is required to prevent making the bleeding worse. Packing is a useful trick to apply prolonged pressure to bleeding veins.

Capillary bleeding or oozing can be helped by diathermy or sutures, but for larger areas it is best controlled by pressure or packing. Haemostatic sprays (e.g. fibrin glue), or biodegradable haemostatic gauze patches (e.g. Surgicel™) are also available.

What other measures are available to reduce operative blood loss?

Following major operative bleeding it is necessary to check the patient's haemoglobin and clotting. Anaemic patients should be transfused intra-operatively. Abnormal clotting can be corrected by fresh frozen plasma or platelet administration. Blood salvage devices or cell savers are suction devices which remove blood from the operative field, filter it and heparinise it to prevent clotting so it can be re-administered to the patient peri or postoperatively.

ALL OPERATIVE BLEEDING SHOULD BE CONTROLLED BEFORE A WOUND IS CLOSED.

13. Reactive haemorrhage, secondary haemorrhage and occult bleeding

What is reactive haemorrhage and how is it controlled?

Reactive haemorrhage is postoperative bleeding in the first few hours after surgery. There are various mechanisms to explain this:

♦ Patient warming up after surgery causing vasodilation.
♦ Blood vessel recovery from peri-operative spasm.
♦ Blood pressure increases as the patient recovers from anaesthesia or due to postoperative pain.
♦ Patient begins moving, coughing or straining following recovery, dislodging clots or sutures.

Initial management involves pressure over the bleeding area and stabilising the patient with intravenous fluids. Correct any clotting abnormalities. Postoperative pain and hypertension should be treated. If these measures fail to control the bleeding the wound should be re-explored and definitive haemostasis achieved.

What is secondary haemorrhage and how is it controlled?

Secondary haemorrhage is postoperative bleeding several days after initial surgery. It is usually caused by necrosis of an area of blood vessel, related to previous repair and is often precipitated by wound infections. It can also be caused by displacement of a blood clot, 'slipping' of a ligature, or erosion around a vascular suture. These phenomena may be precipitated by increased patient mobility.

The principles of management are as for reactive haemorrhage. Re-exploration of the wound, however, may be more hazardous at this time following definitive surgery, and primary repair of the bleeding vessel is more difficult. It may be possible to ligate the vessel, proximally and remotely from the bleeding wound.

3.11.13

What do you understand by occult haemorrhage?

Occult haemorrhage is the term used to describe the situation where there is evidence of ongoing bleeding (tachycardia, hypotension, anaemia) but no obvious external source. The commonest cause is unrecognised intra-abdominal bleeding, but it can occur with bleeding into the chest, into drains or even into the bed or onto the floor.

How does a surgeon calculate blood loss during an operation?

Volumes of blood in the theatre suction device are measured and recorded. Blood-soaked swabs can be weighed. Blood loss can also be estimated from central pressure and haemoglobin concentration. Do not forget to allow for other fluids lost, e.g. urine output and insensible losses (see section 3.10.5).

14. Shock

What is shock and how is it classified?

3.11.14

Shock is an abnormality of the circulatory system that results in a situation where the body's metabolic and oxygen requirements cannot be met. It is not defined solely by blood pressure criteria and there is no laboratory test for it. It is recognised by the clinical manifestations of inadequate organ perfusion and oxygenation, such as pallor, confusion, tachycardia, tachypnoea, and oliguria. The causes of shock can be classified as.

◆ Hypovolaemic - haemorrhage, fistulae, vomiting, pancreatitis, burns.
◆ Distributive - septic, anaphylactic, neurogenic.
◆ Cardiac - cardiogenic.
◆ Obstructive - cardiac tamponade, tension pneumothorax.

Haemorrhagic shock can be classified based on the estimated amount of blood lost. This can be useful in understanding shock and appreciating the symptoms and signs but should not be used to prescribe fluid resuscitation. This should always be directed by the patient's response to fluid therapy.

Table 1. Classification of shock.

	Class I	Class II	Class III	Class IV
Blood loss (ml)	up to 750	750-1500	1500-2000	>2000
Blood loss (%) blood volume	up to 15%	15-30%	30-40%	>40%
Pulse (bpm)	<100	100-120	120-140 weak	>140 weak
Blood pressure	normal	normal	reduced	reduced
Pulse pressure	normal or increased	reduced	reduced	reduced
Respiratory rate (bpm)	14-20	20-30	30-40	>35
Urine output (ml/hr)	>30	20-30	5-15	nil
Mental status	alert	anxious	drowsy	drowsy or unconscious

What is the management of shock?

Always follow the ABC protocol:

◆ A. The Airway - assess and treat any problems immediately before progressing to B.

◆ B. Breathing - assess, and correct if any problems are found; then recheck the airway. Having rechecked the airway, recheck breathing before progressing to C.

◆ C. Circulation - fully assess the circulation and as before, correct any problems, and go back to check the airway, breathing and then back to circulation.

This is a safe system of managing shock. It is also imperative that, whatever the finding in the circulation assessment, two large-bore cannulae must be placed and warmed intravenous fluids given.

Hypovolaemic shock is treated by restoration of circulating blood volume and arresting ongoing bleeding. This may require surgery or interventional radiology

Septic shock is managed by resuscitation as outlined as above, plus large dose intravenous broad-spectrum antibiotics, invasive monitoring and vasopressors if necessary.

Anaphylactic shock requires exactly the same protocol as outlined above, plus intramuscular adrenaline 500 micrograms. This can be repeated as required; corticosteroids and bronchodilators are also given.

The management of shock requires a team approach with surgeons, anaesthetists and radiologists, but the initial few minutes may be the period which determines the final outcome and it is in this period that the management is simple and structured; ABC does not require any thought but is often done poorly.

15. Urinary retention

Why do some patients develop postoperative urinary retention?

The inability to void in the postoperative period is most common in men with pre-existing prostatic hypertrophy. It occurs after lower abdominal surgery, e.g. inguinal hernia repair, or after removing the urethral catheter following other procedures. It may present with lower abdominal pain and distension, and the inability to pass urine. Occasionally it may present as postoperative distress or confusion.

How do you differentiate between postoperative oliguria or anuria, and retention?

If the patient already has a catheter *in situ*, they cannot be in retention unless the catheter is blocked. Try flushing the catheter. If there is no catheter, retention is diagnosed clinically or with an ultrasound bladder scanner.

What is the management of urinary retention in the short and medium term?

Immediate management involves taking a brief urological history, examination of the abdomen and a check of the observation charts. The bladder can be scanned to confirm the patient is in retention. Occasionally retention can be relieved by simple measures such as the sound of running water or a warm bath. When this fails a urethral catheter is passed (see section 2.7.4).

Consider referral to a urologist. Avoid difficult catheterisations if you are not qualified to do so.

16. Postoperative jaundice

What are the common causes of postoperative jaundice?

Jaundice (hyperbilirubinaemia) is clinically recognisable when the serum bilirubin is greater than 40µmol/l. It is classified as pre-hepatic, hepatic or post-hepatic:

◆ Pre-hepatic causes: massive transfusion, residual haematoma, haemolysis.
◆ Hepatocellular causes: drugs (e.g. halothane), alcohol, viral, sepsis and congenital (e.g. Gilbert's disease).
◆ Post-hepatic causes: cholestasis (e.g. residual stones), iatrogenic (e.g. bile duct injuries), tumour.

3.11.16

How can you determine the cause?

◆ History - alcohol, family history, drugs, contacts.
◆ Examination - stools and urine, signs of liver disease, hepatosplenomegaly, palpable gallbladder.
◆ Investigations - screening for hepatitis A, B, C, liver function tests, ultrasound, ERCP, MRCP/CT, liver biopsy.

Why is fluid management particularly important in jaundiced patients?

These patients are difficult to manage because they have complex pathophysiological problems. The liver failure disrupts the body's normal water metabolism leading to high total body sodium and water levels with low potassium levels, in spite of low circulating volume and hyponatraemia. Low serum protein causing peripheral oedema exacerbates the problem.

Inadequate fluid can lead to hepatorenal syndrome. This involves active renal vasoconstriction which reduces renal perfusion causing oliguria and fluid retention. The cause is unknown but is thought to be due to an imbalance between peripheral vasodilators and renal vasoconstrictors. The treatment is difficult because although volume expanders like albumin work, their effect is transitory and isotonic saline is retained in the interstitial fluid worsening ascites and pulmonary oedema.

Rapid fluid resuscitation can lead to pulmonary oedema and heart failure, as well as a risk of rupturing oesophageal varices. Over-enthusiastic correction of hyponatraemia can cause central pontine myelinolysis.

17. Compartment syndrome

What is compartment syndrome and how is it caused?

Compartment syndrome is due to an increase in pressure in the tissues, causing swelling and tissue damage. It is commonest and best described

3.11.17

in the lower limb, where the tissues (muscles) are divided into the compartments of the leg by intermuscular septae, the interosseous membrane, and surrounded by the deep fascia of the leg. The compartments of the lower leg are the extensor compartment, lateral (peroneal) compartment, and deep and superficial posterior compartments.

Compartment syndrome can occur following reperfusion of ischaemic limbs, fractures, crush injuries and burns.

Upper limb compartment syndrome is rare and may follow fractures and ischaemia-reperfusion injury. Abdominal compartment syndrome is a separate condition due to raised intra-abdominal pressure following laparotomy for ischaemic bowel, aneurysm repair, pancreatitis, etc.

How is the diagnosis made?

This is essentially a clinical diagnosis based on a high index of suspicion. Symptoms and signs include severe pain (often out of proportion to the condition or injury), muscle weakness and tenderness, and sensory loss. Absent peripheral pulses, paralysis and a pale, cold limb are late signs. The diagnosis can be confirmed by measurement of the intra-compartmental pressure, with a needle and pressure transducer. A pressure of greater than 30 mmHg is indicative of compartment syndrome.

What is the treatment?

The compartment(s) can be decompressed by performing a fasciotomy: dividing the deep fascia over the compartments to relieve the pressure. The wounds are left open and dressed as they cannot be re-closed immediately due to the swelling. The wounds are then closed at a later stage (delayed primary closure or skin grafting).

Abdominal compartment syndrome is treated by reopening the abdomen and leaving it open with dressings or a sterile plastic seal over the abdominal contents. The abdomen can be re-closed at a later stage.

What are the complications?

Long-term sequelae of inadequately treated compartment syndrome include muscle wasting and nerve injury, e.g. foot drop, if the lateral compartment of the leg is involved, or Volkmann's ischaemic contracture of the arm.

Chapter 12

Late complications, discharge and follow-up

1. Postoperative confusion

What are the causes of postoperative confusion?

Pre-operative factors:

- Old age.
- Change of environment.
- Diabetes.
- Pre-operative drug and alcohol dependency states.
- Pre-existing depression or dementia.
- Concomitant medical conditions, such as previous cerebral, cardiac, pulmonary or renal disorders.

Operative factors:

- Major surgery.
- Major blood loss.
- General anaesthesia.

3.12.1

Postoperative factors:

◆ Anaemia.
◆ Hypotension.
◆ Pain.
◆ Central: meningitis, tumour, stroke and post-ictal.
◆ Drugs: especially anaesthetic agents, tranquilisers, benzodiazepines.
◆ Infections: chest, urine, wound, septicaemia.
◆ Respiratory: hypoxia.
◆ Urinary retention.
◆ Metabolic: hyponatraemia, hypo- or hyperglycaemia, hypocalcaemia, alcohol withdrawal, uraemia, thyroid disturbance, liver failure, diabetes.

Postoperative confusion is a type of acute confusional state. It is potentially dangerous to assume that it is just a result of surgery, as life-threatening abnormalities, such as hypoxia, may be overlooked. The most common cause of a postoperative acute confusional state is pre-existing dementia, often sub-clinical, combined with the effects of the anaesthetic agents and change of environment.

What is the management of postoperative acute confusional state?

◆ A full history and examination is essential.
◆ Investigations: pulse, blood pressure, respiratory rate, temperature, blood glucose, oxygen saturation, electrolytes, thyroid and liver function tests, blood gases and infection screen.
◆ Treat the cause.
◆ Very judicious use of tranquilisers.
◆ Never assume the patient is 'just confused'; always exclude life-threatening causes.

2. Psychological effects of surgery

What are the possible psychological effects of surgery?

Psychological problems after surgery are common and include confusion, anxiety and depression. They depend on the patient's pre-operative well-being, personality type and the way in which they react to life-changing events. Other important factors include the type of surgery and the occurrence of unexpected events or complications.

All patients have some pre-operative stress and anxiety, but for some the fear may be so great it prevents them from being able to undergo essential surgery. Conversely, the patient may have been waiting for a long time for an operation they hope will improve their life and so may be excited and elated. Awareness during the operation has been shown to have negative psychological effects. Procedures which may cause severe deformity or disability, e.g. mastectomy, amputation and extensive facial surgery, may cause depression and low self esteem, often associated with withdrawal from society. Cosmetic procedures can improve patients' psychological well being.

The psychological effect of surgery on children is often more severe than adults and can have long-term effects, especially if it involves multiple procedures and long hospital stays or causes disability or disfigurement.

What resources are available to help with psychological distress?

Most hospitals have psychologists, psychiatrists and counsellors available. However, all personnel involved in the care of surgical patients require some understanding of the psychological effects of surgery. This enables expert help to be arranged before any psychological ill effects of surgery can escalate.

Which patients are at greatest risk of postoperative psychological problems?

Patients with pre-existing psychological problems, in particular, body dysmorphic disorders and personality disorders, are at risk of reacting badly to surgery generally. Some procedures seem to cause particularly high psychological morbidity. This may be because they seem to appeal to patients who have psychological problems, e.g. female genitoplasty and cosmetic facial surgery, especially in young 'normal' looking people.

What is meant by institutionalisation in relation to hospitals?

This term refers to people, usually the elderly or disabled who, due to a combination of a prolonged hospital admission, and poor management, become so dependent on the hospital (the institution) for their physical care and psychological wellbeing, that it becomes impossible for them or their carers to imagine that they could exist in their pre-hospital environment, even when they are as physically well as they were prior to the illness which led to their admission.

3. Pressure sores

How do pressures sores develop?

3.12.3

Pressure sores (decubitus ulcers) are ulcers due to ischaemia and tissue damage, secondary to prolonged pressure on an area of skin. The affected area is compressed so there is inadequate blood supply to the local skin and subcutaneous tissues, leading to infarction, necrosis and ulceration.

Pressure sores commonly occur over the sacrum and heels of patients on prolonged bedrest, but can occur on the occiput, shoulders, elbows, buttocks or toes.

What is pressure area care?

Pressure area care is a system devised to prevent pressure sores. Simple measures include padding (Gelfoam® or polo cushions) to prevent heel ulceration, bed cradles to prevent toe pressure sores by compression from bedclothes, and frequent turning and repositioning of patients to prevent sacral pressure area sores. Special beds with soft mattresses or variable load distribution are also available. Adequate nutrition, early mobilisation, relief of ischaemic extremities etc., are also important.

What groups are at high risk of pressure sores?

◆   General factors: old age, immobility, malnutrition, obesity, bedrest, malignancy, dementia, diabetes.
◆   Local factors: ischaemic extremities, neuropathies, infections.

What are the long-term consequences?

Delayed discharge, delayed mobilisation, wound and pressure area infection, pneumonia, death.

4. Rehabilitation

What is postoperative rehabilitation?

Rehabilitation is the process of restoration of skills by a person who has had an illness, injury or operation, so as to gain maximum self-sufficiency and to function in a normal, or as near normal manner as possible, i.e. to achieve their maximum potential quality of life postoperatively.

3.12.4

Why is rehabilitation important?

Rehabilitation is important to fulfil patient expectations, and to facilitate early, safe discharge. Rehabilitation should be planned pre-operatively in a multi-disciplinary environment. Surgery can be wasted by failing to help the patient rehabilitate.

What groups of patients benefit most?

Following major surgery, maximum benefit is achieved in the elderly, those with poor social support, patients with physical or mental incapacity and those who have suffered psychological distress.

Who is involved?

Rehabilitation is best performed using a team approach.

This involves specialists in:

◆ Rehabilitation medicine, e.g. prosthetics departments.
◆ Physiotherapy - to optimise mobility (see section 3.12.5).
◆ Occupational therapy, e.g. kitchen skills, toilet skills.
◆ Social services - for organizing home helps, meals on wheels, etc.
◆ Psychology.
◆ Psychiatry.
◆ General practice.

5. Physiotherapy

What is the role of the physiotherapist in postoperative care?

3.12.5

Physiotherapy is an important part of the rehabilitation process. Physiotherapy care starts with a full pre-operative assessment, including medical and social history, details of level of mobility, patient expectations and an explanation of protocols. Postoperative mobility problems and discharge planning should be discussed at this stage.

Early postoperative care includes chest physio, exercises for muscle groups affected by surgery, restoration of mobility and psychological support. Chest physio is predominantly aimed at preventing postoperative atelectasis and chest infections in patients following thoracic or abdominal surgery, or those with pre-existing respiratory disease. It involves breathing exercises, chest percussion, manual vibration techniques and patient education regarding methods of clearing retained secretions.

Muscle group exercises are particularly important following orthopaedic and peripheral vascular surgery. Active and passive muscle contraction is encouraged by specific exercises, designed to mobilise and strengthen specific muscle groups, prevent muscle imbalance and prevent contractures.

Restoration of mobility is a complicated series of manoeuvres designed to give confidence, restore core stability and build up strength for walking and transfers (bed/chair, chair/toilet, etc.). It is especially important following orthopaedic back/hip/knee surgery, vascular lower limb reconstructions and amputations.

Late postoperative physio is a continuation of this process, and involves gym-work, parallel bars and other specific procedures for particular patient groups, e.g. wheelchair mobility and transfers for paraplegic patients, oedema control and PAMAID (prosthetic post-amputation mobility aid) for amputees.

Physiotherapists should contribute to pre-operative planning at multi-disciplinary meetings and be involved with rehabilitation teams in discharge planning, ongoing care and patient education. Physiotherapy may continue after discharge on an outpatient basis, especially for sports injury rehabilitation and walking programs for claudicants, etc.

6. Palliative care

What is palliative care?

3.12.6

Palliative care is given to improve the quality of life of patients who have an incurable, serious or life-threatening, usually terminal disease. The goal of palliative care is to prevent or treat as early as possible the symptoms of the disease, side effects caused by treatment of the disease, and psychological, social, and spiritual problems related to the disease or its treatment.

What is palliative surgery?

Palliative surgery does not treat the underlying disease, but is done to control symptoms of the disease, such as pain, bowel obstruction or incontinence.

What is a palliative care team and who would be involved?

The palliative care team is a dedicated multi-disciplinary team who use their expertise to help patients and their families maintain their maximum physical and emotional potential usually in a terminal care situation. They not only provide help with pain and symptom control but provide psychological, social and spiritual support as well. The team comprises a core of doctors, nurses, and administrative staff but the extended team also includes occupational therapists, dietitians, physiotherapists, speech and language therapists, clinical psychologists, social workers and religious representatives such as priests and rabbis.

What is the role of a hospice?

A hospice is an establishment for the provision of terminal care. It includes an inpatient facility and extended care into the community. It is usually staffed by a palliative care team.

7. Discharge

What are the fundamental requirements before a patient can be discharged from hospital?

A patient is ready for discharge when a clinical decision is made that the patient is ready for discharge and the patient is safe to discharge/transfer.

What are the common delays to discharge?

- Awaiting nursing or residential placement.
- Awaiting assessment of needs.
- Awaiting further NHS care.
- Awaiting placement of patient's choice.
- Awaiting public funding.
- Awaiting domiciliary care.

What can be done to reduce delays?

Multi-disciplinary decisions made early, recognise potential problems early and try to pre-empt causes of delay. Involve the discharge team if the hospital has one.

What is a discharge summary?

It is a transfer of care form detailing the patient's condition, surgery, recovery, any significant complications or alteration, especially in medications. Also included are a list of medications and advice on whether the general practitioner should continue them, details of follow-up and any community care required and arrangements made. A copy is sent to the general practitioner, one is filed in the hospital notes, and further copies are sent to the patient, palliative care teams, district nurses etc., if appropriate.

8. Surgery and the law

3.12.8

Outline the legal requirements for a case of negligence to arise against a doctor

Negligence arises when one person owes to another a duty of care and breaches that duty, and reasonably foreseeable harm arises as a result of that breach. Medical negligence is the failure of a healthcare provider to treat and care for a patient with a reasonable degree of skill and care. Legal negligence requires the triad of duty, breach and damage.

Describe what you understand in legal terms by an incompetent practitioner

An incompetent practitioner is one who falls below recognised standards of care.

When are breaches of confidence mandatory?

When a court of law requires it, if there is a case of notifiable diseases, if it is required for use as evidence in a healthcare tribunal and when the patient is suspected of terrorism.

When are they discretionary?

If maintaining confidentiality may put the patient at significant risk, or if it may place others at risk through criminal activity.

Informed consent

(See section 1.3.9).

Index

A

E

F

G